DIETARY GUIDE

DIETARY GUIDE

ALBERT O. GOMBER
EDITOR

Novinka Books

For permission to use material from this book please contact us:
Telephone 631-231-7269; Fax 631-231-8175
Web Site: http://www.novapublishers.com

NOTICE TO THE READER

The Publisher has taken reasonable care in the preparation of this book, but makes no expressed or implied warranty of any kind and assumes no responsibility for any errors or omissions. No liability is assumed for incidental or consequential damages in connection with or arising out of information contained in this book. The Publisher shall not be liable for any special, consequential, or exemplary damages resulting, in whole or in part, from the readers' use of, or reliance upon, this material.

Independent verification should be sought for any data, advice or recommendations contained in this book. In addition, no responsibility is assumed by the publisher for any injury and/or damage to persons or property arising from any methods, products, instructions, ideas or otherwise contained in this publication.

This publication is designed to provide accurate and authoritative information with regard to the subject matter covered herein. It is sold with the clear understanding that the Publisher is not engaged in rendering legal or any other professional services. If legal or any other expert assistance is required, the services of a competent person should be sought. FROM A DECLARATION OF PARTICIPANTS JOINTLY ADOPTED BY A COMMITTEE OF THE AMERICAN BAR ASSOCIATION AND A COMMITTEE OF PUBLISHERS.

Library of Congress Cataloging-in-Publication Data:
Available Upon Request

ISBN 1-59454-654-1

Published by Nova Science Publishers, Inc. New York

CONTENTS

PREFACE

This book is excerpted from 'The Dietary Guidelines for Americans [Dietary Guidelines]' and augmented with a full index and a list of questions and answers related to guidelines for diet. It contains science-based advice to promote health and to reduce risk for major chronic diseases through diet and physical activity. Major causes of morbidity and mortality in the United States are related to poor diet and a sedentary lifestyle. Some specific diseases linked to poor diet and physical inactivity include cardiovascular disease, type 2 diabetes, hypertension, osteoporosis, and certain cancers. Furthermore, poor diet and physical inactivity, resulting in an energy imbalance (more calories consumed than expended), are the most important factors contributing to the increase in overweight and obesity.

In: Dietary Guide
Editor: Albert O. Gomber, pp. 1-10

ISBN: 1-59454-654-1
© 2007 Nova Science Publishers, Inc.

EXECUTIVE SUMMARY

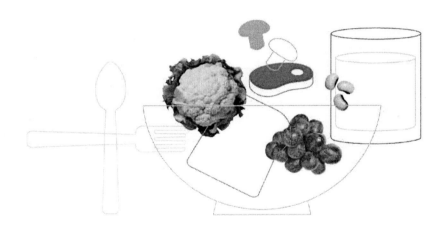

The *Dietary Guidelines for Americans [Dietary Guidelines]* provides science-based advice to promote health and to reduce risk for major chronic diseases through diet and physical activity. Major causes of morbidity and mortality in the United States are related to poor diet and a sedentary lifestyle. Some specific diseases linked to poor diet and physical inactivity include cardiovascular disease, type 2 diabetes, hypertension, osteoporosis, and certain cancers. Furthermore, poor diet and physical inactivity, resulting in an energy imbalance (more calories consumed than expended), are the most important factors contributing to the increase in overweight and obesity in this country. Combined with physical activity, following a diet that does not provide excess calories according to the recommendations in this document should enhance the health of most individuals.

An important component of each 5-year revision of the *Dietary Guidelines* is the analysis of new scientific information by the Dietary Guidelines Advisory Committee (DGAC) appointed by the Secretaries of the U.S. Department of Health and Human Services (HHS) and the U.S. Department of Agriculture (USDA). This analysis, published in the DGAC Report (http://www.health.gov/dietaryguidelines/dga2005/ report/), is the primary resource for development of the report on the Guidelines by the Departments. The *Dietary Guidelines* and the report of the DGAC differ in scope and purpose compared to reports for previous versions of the *Guidelines*. The 2005 DGAC report is a detailed scientific analysis. The scientific report was used to develop the *Dietary Guidelines* jointly between the two Departments and forms the basis of recommendations that will be used by USDA and HHS for program and policy development.

Thus it is a publication oriented toward policymakers, nutrition educators, nutritionists, and healthcare providers rather than to the general public, as with previous versions of the *Dietary Guidelines*, and contains more technical information.

The intent of the *Dietary Guidelines* is to summarize and synthesize knowledge regarding individual nutrients and food components into recommendations for a pattern of eating that can be adopted by the public. In this publication, Key Recommendations are grouped under nine inter-related focus areas. The recommendations are based on the preponderance of scientific evidence for lowering risk of chronic disease and promoting health. It is important to remember that these are integrated messages that should be implemented as a whole. Taken together, they encourage most Americans to eat fewer calories, be more active, and make wiser food choices.

A basic premise of the *Dietary Guidelines* is that nutrient needs should be met primarily through consuming foods. Foods provide an array of nutrients and other compounds that may have beneficial effects on health. In certain cases, fortified foods and dietary supplements may be useful sources of one or more nutrients that otherwise might be consumed in less than recommended amounts. However, dietary supplements, while recommended in some cases, cannot replace a healthful diet.

Two examples of eating patterns that exemplify the *Dietary Guidelines* are the USDA Food Guide (http:// www.usda.gov/cnpp/pyramid.html) and the DASH (Dietary Approaches to Stop Hypertension) Eating Plan.[1] Both of these eating patterns are designed to integrate dietary recommendations into a healthy way to eat for most individuals. These eating patterns are not weight loss diets, but rather illustrative examples of how to eat in accordance with the *Dietary Guidelines*. Both eating patterns are constructed across a range of calorie levels to meet the needs of various age and gender groups. For the USDA Food Guide, nutrient content estimates for each food group and subgroup are based on population- weighted food intakes. Nutrient content estimates for the DASH Eating Plan are based on selected foods chosen for a sample 7-day menu. While originally developed to study the effects of an eating pattern on the prevention and treatment of hypertension, DASH is one example of a balanced eating plan consistent with the 2005 *Dietary Guidelines*.

Taken together, [the Dietary Guidelines] encourage most Americans to eat fewer calories, be more active, and make wiser food choices.

Throughout most of this publication, examples use a 2,000-calorie level as a reference for consistency with the Nutrition Facts Panel. Although this level is used as a reference, recommended calorie intake will differ for individuals based on age, gender, and activity level. At each calorie level, individuals who eat nutrient-dense foods may be able to meet their recommended nutrient intake without consuming their full calorie allotment. The remaining calories — *discretionary calorie allowance* individuals flexibility to consume some foods and beverages that may contain added fats, added sugars, and alcohol.

The recommendations in the *Dietary Guidelines* are for Americans over 2 years of age. It is important to incorporate the food preferences of different racial/ethnic groups, vege-tarians, and other groups when planning diets and developing educational programs and materials. The USDA Food Guide and the DASH Eating Plan are flexible enough to accommodate a range of food preferences and cuisines.

The *Dietary Guidelines* is intended primarily for use by policymakers, healthcare providers, nutritionists, and nutrition educators. The information in the *Dietary Guidelines* is useful for the development of educational materials and aids policymakers in designing and implementing nutrition-related programs, including federal food, nutrition education, and information programs. In addition, this publication has the potential to provide authoritative statements as provided for in the Food and Drug

Administration Modernization Act (FDAMA). Because the *Dietary Guidelines* contains discussions where the science is emerging, only statements included in the Executive Summary and the sections titled "Key recommendations," which reflect the preponderance of scientific evidence, can be used for identification of authoritative statements. The recommendations are interrelated and mutually dependent; thus the statements in this document should be used together in the context of planning an overall healthful diet. However, even following just some of the recommendations can have health benefits.

The following is a listing of the *Dietary Guidelines* by chapter.

ADEQUATE NUTRIENTS WITHIN CALORIE NEEDS

Key Recommendations

- Consume a variety of nutrient-dense foods and beverages within and among the basic food groups while choosing foods that limit the intake of saturated and *trans* fats, cholesterol, added sugars, salt, and alcohol.
- Meet recommended intakes within energy needs byadopting a balanced eating pattern, such as the USDA Food Guide or the DASH Eating Plan.

Key Recommendations for Specific Population Groups

- *People over age 50.* Consume vitamin B12 in its crystalline form (i.e., fortified foods or supplements).
- *Women of childbearing age who may become pregnant.* Eat foods high in heme-iron and/or consume iron-rich plant foods or iron-fortified foods with an enhancer of iron absorption, such as vitamin C-rich foods.
- *Women of childbearing age who may become pregnant and those in the first trimester of pregnancy.* Consume adequate synthetic folic acid daily (from fortified foods or supplements) in addition to food forms of folate from a varied diet.
- *Older adults, people with dark skin, and people exposed to insufficient ultraviolet band radiation (i.e.,sunlight).* Consume extra vitamin D from vitamin D-fortified foods and/or supplements.

WEIGHT MANAGEMENT

Key Recommendations

- To maintain body weight in a healthy range balance calories from foods and beverages with calories expended.
- To prevent gradual weight gain over time, make small decreases in food and beverage calories and increase physical activity.

Key Recommendations for Specific Population Groups

- *Those who need to lose weight.* Aim for a slow, steady weight loss by decreasing calorie intake while maintaining an adequate nutrient intake and increasing physical activity.
- *Overweight children.* Reduce the rate of body weight gain while allowing growth and development. Consult a healthcare provider before placing a child on a weight-reduction diet
- *Pregnant women.* Ensure appropriate weight gain as specified by a healthcare provider.
- *Breastfeeding women.* Moderate weight reduction Meet recommended intakes within energy needs by is safe and does not compromise weight gain of the nursing infant.
- *Overweight adults and overweight children with chronic diseases and/or on medication.* Consult a healthcare provider about weight loss strategies prior to starting a weight-reduction program to ensure appropriate management of other health conditions.

PHYSICAL ACTIVITY

Key Recommendations

- Engage in regular physical activity and reduce sedentary activities to promote health, psychological well-being, and a healthy body weight.

  - To reduce the risk of chronic disease in adulthood: Engage in at least 30 minutes of moderate-intensity physical activity, above usual activity, at work or home on most days of the week.

- For most people, greater health benefits can be obtained by engaging in physical activity of more vigorous intensity or longer duration.
- To help manage body weight and prevent gradual, unhealthy body weight gain in adulthood: Engage in approximately 60 minutes of moderate- to vigorous- intensity activity on most days of the week while not exceeding caloric intake requirements.
- To sustain weight loss in adulthood: Participate in at least 60 to 90 minutes of daily moderate-intensity physical activity while not exceeding caloric intake requirements. Some people may need to consult with a healthcare provider before participating in this level of activity.

- Achieve physical fitness by including cardiovascular conditioning, stretching exercises for flexibility, and resistance exercises or calisthenics for muscle strength and endurance.

Key Recommendations for Specific Population Groups

- *Children and adolescents.* Engage in at least 60 minutes of physical activity on most, preferably all, days of the week.
- *Pregnant women.* In the absence of medical or obstetric complications, incorporate 30 minutes or more of moderate-intensity physical activity on most, if not all, days of the week. Avoid activities with a high risk of falling or abdominal trauma.
- *Breastfeeding women.* Be aware that neither acute nor regular exercise adversely affects the mother's ability to successfully breastfeed.
- *Older adults.* Participate in regular physical activity to reduce functional declines associated with aging and to achieve the other benefits of physical activity identified for all adults.

FOOD GROUPS TO ENCOURAGE

Key Recommendations

- Consume a sufficient amount of fruits and vegetables while staying within energy needs. Two cups of fruit and 2½ cups of vegetables per day are recommended for a reference 2,000-calorie intake, with higher or : lower amounts depending on the calorie level.

- Choose a variety of fruits and vegetables each day. In particular, select from all five vegetable subgroups (dark green, orange, legumes, starchy vegetables, and other vegetables) several times a week.
- Consume 3 or more ounce-equivalents of whole-grain products per day, with the rest of the recommended grains coming from enriched or whole-grain products. In general, at least half the grains should come from whole grains.
- Consume 3 cups per day of fat-free or low-fat milk or equivalent milk products.

Key Recommendations for Specific Population Groups

- *Children and adolescents.* Consume whole-grain products often; at least half the grains should be whole grains. Children 2 to 8 years should consume 2 cups per day of fat-free or low-fat milk or equivalent milk Achieve physical fitness by including cardiovascular products. Children 9 years of age and older should consume 3 cups per day of fat-free or low-fat milk or equivalent milk products.

FATS

Key Recommendations

- Consume less than 10 percent of calories from saturated fatty acids and less than 300 mg/day of cholesterol, and keep *trans* fatty acid consumption as low as possible.
- Keep total fat intake between 20-35 percent of calories, with most fats coming from sources of polyun-saturated and monounsaturated fatty acids, such as fish, nuts, and vegetable oils.
- When selecting and preparing meat, poultry, dry beans, and milk or milk products, make choices that are lean, low-fat, or fat-free.
- Limit intake of fats and oils high in saturated and/or *trans* fatty acids, and choose products low in such fats and oils.

Key Recommendations for Specific Population Groups

- *Children and adolescents.* Keep total fat intake between 30 to 35 percent of calories for children 2 to 3 years of age and between 25 to 35 percent of calories for children and adolescents 4 to 18 years of age, with most fats coming from sources of polyunsaturated and monounsaturated fatty acids, such as fish, nuts, and vegetable oils.

CARBOHYDRATES

Key Recommendations

- Choose fiber-rich fruits, vegetables, and whole grains often.
- Choose and prepare foods and beverages with little added sugars or caloric sweeteners, such as amounts suggested by the USDA Food Guide and the DASH Eating Plan.
- Reduce the incidence of dental caries by practicing good oral hygiene and consuming sugar- and starch-containing foods and beverages less frequently.

SODIUM AND POTASSIUM

Key Recommendations

- Consume less than 2,300 mg (approximately 1 tsp of salt) of sodium per day.
- Choose and prepare foods with little salt. At the same time, consume potassium-rich foods, such as fruits and vegetables.

Key Recommendations for Specific Population Groups

- *Individuals with hypertension, blacks, and middle-aged and older adults.* Aim to consume no more than 1,500 mg of sodium per day, and meet the potassium recommendation (4,700 mg/day) with food.

ALCOHOLIC BEVERAGES

Key Recommendations

▪ Those who choose to drink alcoholic beverages should do so sensibly and in moderation – defined as the consumption of up to one drink per day for women and up to two drinks per day for men.

▪ Alcoholic beverages should not be consumed by some individuals, including those who cannot restrict their alcohol intake, women of childbearing age who may become pregnant, pregnant and lactating women, children and adolescents, individuals taking medications that can interact with alcohol, and those with specific medical conditions.

▪ Alcoholic beverages should be avoided by individuals engaging in activities that require attention, skill, or coordination, such as driving or operating machinery.

FOOD SAFETY

Key Recommendations

▪ To avoid microbial foodborne illness:
  ▪ Clean hands, food contact surfaces and fruits and vegetable. Meat and poultry should not be washed or rinsed
  ▪ Separate raw, cooked and ready-to-eat foods while shopping, preparing or storing foods.
  ▪ Cook foods to a safe temperature to kill microorganisms
  ▪ Chill (refrigerate) perishable food promptly and defrost foods properly.
  ▪ Avoid raw (unpasteurized) milk or any products made from unpasteurized milk, raw or partially cooked eggs or foods containing raw eggs, raw or undercooked meat and poultry, unpasteurized juices, and raw sprouts

Key Recommendations for Specific Population Groups

▪ *Infants and young children,pregnant women,older adults,and those who are immunocompromised.* Do not eat or drink raw (unpasteurized) milk or any products made from unpasteurized milk, raw or partially cooked eggs or foods containing raw eggs, raw or undercooked meat and poultry, raw or undercooked fish or shellfish, unpasteurized juices, and raw sprouts.

▪ *Pregnant women, older adults, and those who are immunocompromised:* Only eat certain deli meats and frankfurters that have been reheated to steaming hot. Those who choose to drink alcoholic beverages should

REFERENCES

[1] NIH Publication No. 03-4082, Facts about the DASH Eating Plan, United States Department of Health and Human Services, National Institutes of Health, National Heart, Lung, and Blood Institute, Karanja NM et al. *Journal of the American Dietetic Association (JADA)* **8**:S19-27, 1999. http://www.nhlbi.nih.gov/health/public/ heart/hbp/dash/.

In: Dietary Guide   ISBN: 1-59454-654-1
Editor: Albert O. Gomber, pp. 11-17   © 2007 Nova Science Publishers, Inc.

Chapter 1

BACKGROUND AND PURPOSE OF THE DIETARY GUIDELINES FOR AMERICANS

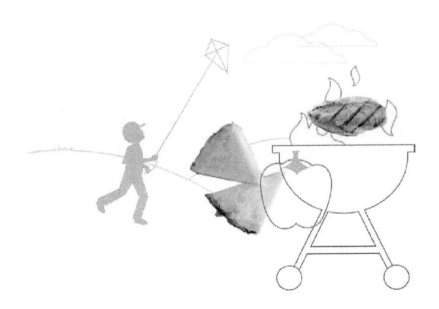

The *Dietary Guidelines for Americans [Dietary Guidelines],* first published in 1980, provides science-based advice to promote health and to reduce risk for chronic diseases through diet and physical activity. The recommendations contained within the *Dietary Guidelines* are targeted to the general public over 2 years of age who are living in the United States. Because of its focus on health promotion and risk reduction, the *Dietary Guidelines* form the basis of federal food, nutrition education, and information programs.

By law (Public Law 101-445, Title III, 7 U.S.C. 5301 et seq.), the *Dietary Guidelines* is reviewed, updated if necessary, and published every 5 years. The process to create the *Dietary Guidelines* is a joint effort of the U.S. Department of Health and Human Services (HHS) and the U.S. Department of Agriculture (USDA) and has evolved to include three stages.

In the first stage, an external scientific Advisory Committee appointed by the two Departments conducted an analysis of new scientific information and prepared a report summarizing its findings.[1] The Advisory Committee's report was made available to the public and Government agencies for comment. The Committee's analysis was the primary resource for development of the *Dietary Guidelines* by the Departments. A significant amount of the new scientific information used by the Dietary Guidelines Advisory Committee (DGAC) was based on the Dietary Reference Intake (DRI) reports published since 2000 by the Institute of Medicine (IOM), in particular the macronutrient report and the fluid and electrolyte report.

During the second stage, the Departments jointly developed Key Recommendations based on the Advisory Committee's report and public and agency comments.

The *Dietary Guidelines* details these science-based policy recommend-dations. Finally, in the third stage, the two Departments developed messages communicating the *Dietary Guidelines* to the general public.

Because of the three-part process used to develop and communicate the 2005 *Dietary Guidelines*, this publication and the report of the DGAC differ in scope and purpose compared to reports for previous versions of the *Guidelines*. The 2005 DGAC report is a detailed scientific analysis that identifies key issues such as energy balance, the consequences of a sedentary lifestyle, and the need to emphasize certain food choices to address nutrition issues for the American public. The scientific report was used to develop the *Dietary Guidelines* jointly between the two Departments, and this publication forms the basis of recommendations that will be used by USDA and HHS for program and policy development. Thus it is a publication oriented toward policymakers, nutrition educators, nutritionists and healthcare providers rather than to the general public, as with previous versions of the *Dietary Guidelines*, and contains more technical information.

New sections in the *Dietary Guidelines*, consistent with its use for program development, are a glossary of terms and appendixes with detailed information about the USDA Food Guide and the Dietary Approaches to Stop Hypertension (DASH) Eating Plan as well as tables listing sources of some nutrients. Consumer messages have been developed to educate the public about the Key

Recommendations in the *Dietary Guidelines* and will be used in materials targeted for consumers separate from this publication. In organizing the *Dietary Guidelines* for the Departments, chapters 2 to 10 were given titles that characterize the topic of each section, and the *Dietary Guidelines* itself is presented as an integrated set of Key Recommendations in each topic area.

These Key Recommendations are based on a preponderance of the scientific evidence of nutritional factors that are important for lowering risk of chronic disease and promoting health. To optimize the beneficial impact of these recommendations on health, the *Guidelines* should be implemented in their entirety.

IMPORTANCE OF THE *DIETARY GUIDELINES* FOR HEALTH PROMOTION AND DISEASE PREVENTION

Good nutrition is vital to good health and is absolutely essential for the healthy growth and development of children and adolescents. Major causes of morbidity and mortality in the United States are related to poor diet and a sedentary lifestyle. Specific diseases and conditions linked to poor diet include cardiovascular disease, hypertension, dyslipidemia, type 2 diabetes, overweight and obesity, osteoporosis, constipation, diverticular disease, iron deficiency anemia, oral disease, malnutrition, and some cancers. Lack of physical activity has been associated with cardiovascular disease, hypertension, overweight and obesity, osteoporosis, diabetes, and certain cancers. Furthermore, muscle strengthening and improving balance can reduce falls and increase functional status among older adults. Together with physical activity, a high-quality diet that does not provide excess calories should enhance the health of most individuals.

Poor diet and physical inactivity, resulting in an energy imbalance (more calories consumed than expended), are the most important factors contributing to the increase in overweight and obesity in this country. Moreover, over-weight and obesity are major risk factors for certain chronic diseases such as diabetes. In 1999-2002, 65 percent of U.S. adults were overweight, an increase from 56 percent in 1988– percent of adults were obese, an increase from 23 percent in an earlier survey. Dramatic increases in the prevalence of overweight have occurred in children and adolescents of both sexes, with approximately 16 percent of children and adolescents aged 6 to 19 years considered to be over-weight (1999– [2] In order to reverse this trend, many Americans need to consume fewer calories, be more active, and make wiser choices within and among food groups. The *Dietary Guidelines* provides a framework to promote healthier lifestyles (see ch. 3).

Given the importance of a balanced diet to health, the intent of the *Dietary Guidelines* is to summarize and synthesize knowledge regarding individual nutrients and food components into recommendations for an overall pattern of eating that can be adopted by the general public. These patterns are exemplified by the USDA Food Guide and the DASH Eating Plan (see ch. 2 and app. A). The *Dietary Guidelines* is applicable to the food preferences of different racial/ethnic groups, vegetarians, and other groups. This concept of balanced eating patterns should be utilized in planning diets for various population groups.

There is a growing body of evidence which demonstrates that following a diet that complies with the *Dietary Guidelines* may reduce the risk of chronic disease. Recently, it was reported that dietary patterns consistent with recommended dietary guidance were associated with a lower risk of mortality among individuals age 45 years and older in the United States. [3] The authors of the study estimated that about 16 percent and 9 percent of mortality from any cause in men and women, respectively, could be eliminated by the adoption of desirable dietary behaviors. Currently, adherence to the *Dietary Guidelines* is low among the U.S. population. Data from USDA illustrate the degree of change in the overall dietary pattern of Americans needed to be consistent with a food pattern encouraged by the *Dietary Guidelines* (fig. 1).

A basic premise of the *Dietary Guidelines* is that nutrient needs should be met primarily through consuming foods. Foods provide an array of nutrients (as well as phyto-chemicals, antioxidants, etc.) and other compounds that may have beneficial effects on health. In some cases, fortified foods may be useful sources of one or more nutrients that otherwise might be consumed in less than recommended amounts. Supplements may be useful when they fill a specific identified nutrient gap that cannot or is not otherwise being met by the individual's intake of food. Nutrient supplements cannot replace a healthful diet. Individuals who are already consuming the recommended amount of a nutrient in food will not achieve any additional health benefit if they also take the nutrient as a supplement. In fact, in some cases, supplements and fortified foods may cause intakes to exceed the safe levels of nutrients. Another important premise of the *Dietary Guidelines* is that foods should be prepared and handled in such a way that reduces risk of foodborne illness.

USES OF THE DIETARY GUIDELINES

The *Dietary Guidelines* is intended primarily for use by policymakers, healthcare providers, nutritionists, and nutrition educators. While the *Dietary Guidelines* was developed for healthy Americans 2 years of age and older, where appropriate, the needs of specific population groups have been addressed. In addition, other individuals may find this report helpful in making healthful

choices. As noted previously, the recommendations contained within the *Dietary Guidelines* will aid the public in reducing their risk for obesity and chronic disease. Specific uses of the
Dietary Guidelines include:

Development of Educational Materials and Communications.
The information in the *Dietary Guidelines* is useful for the development of educational materials. For example, the federal dietary guidance-related publications are required by law to be based on the *Dietary Guidelines*. In addition, this publication will guide the development of messages to communicate the *Dietary Guidelines* to the public. Finally, the USDA Food Guide, the food label, and Nutrition Facts Panel provide information that is useful for implementing the key recommendations in the *Dietary Guidelines* and should be integrated into educational and communication messages.

Development of Nutrition-Related Programs.
The *Dietary Guidelines* aids policymakers in designing and implementing nutrition-related programs. The Federal Government bases its nutrition programs, such as the National Child Nutrition Programs or the Elderly Nutrition Program, on the *Dietary Guidelines*.

Development of Authoritative Statements.
The *Dietary Guidelines* has the potential to provide intake of food. authoritative statements as provided for in the Food and Drug Administration Modernization Act (FDAMA). Because the recommendations are interrelated and mutu -ally dependent, the statements in this publication should be used together in the context of an overall healthful diet. Likewise, because the *Dietary Guidelines* contains discussions about emerging science, only statements included in the Executive Summary and the highlighted boxes entitled "Key Recommendations", which reflect the preponderance of scientific evidence, can be used for identification of authoritative statements.

A graphical depiction of the degree of change in average daily food consumption by Americans that would be needed to be consistent with the food patterns encouraged by the *Dietary Guidelines for Americans*. The zero line represents average consumption levels from each food group or subgroup by females 31 to 50 years of age and males 31 to 50 years of age. Bars above the zero line represent recommended increases in food group consumption, while bars below the line represent recommended decreases.

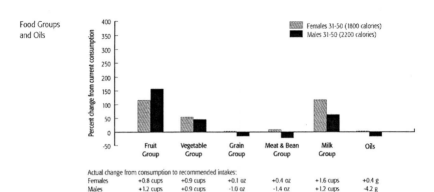

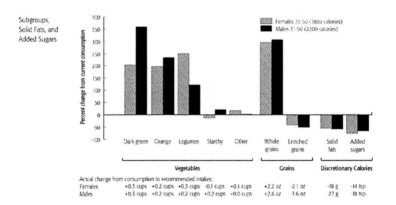

[a] USDA Food Guide in comparison to National Health and Nutrition Examination Survey 20012002 consumption data.

[b] Increases in amounts of some food groups are offset by decreases in amounts of solid fats (i.e., saturated and *trans* fats) and added sugars so that total calorie intake is at the recommended level.

Figure 1. Percent Increase or Decrease From Current Consumption (Zero Line) to Recommended Intakes [a,b]

REFERENCES

[1] For more information about the process, summary data, and the resources used by the Advisory Committee, see the 2005 Dietary Guidelines

Advisory   Committee   Report   (2005   DGAC   Report)   at
http://www.health.gov/dietaryguidelines.

[2] Hedley AA, Ogden CL, Johnson CL, Carroll MD, Curtin LR, Flegal KM.
Prevalence of overweight and obesity among U.S. children, adolescents,
and adults, 1999-2002. *Journal of the American Medical Association
(JAMA)* **291**(23):2847-2850, 2004.

[3] Kant AK, Graubard BI, Schatzkin A. Dietary patterns predict mortality in
a national cohort: The national health interview surveys, 1987 and 1992.
Journal of Nutrition (J Nutr) **134**:1793-1799, 2004.

In: Dietary Guide
Editor: Albert O. Gomber, pp. 19-33

ISBN: 1-59454-654-1
© 2007 Nova Science Publishers, Inc.

Chapter 2

ADEQUATE NUTRIENTS WITHIN CALORIE NEEDS

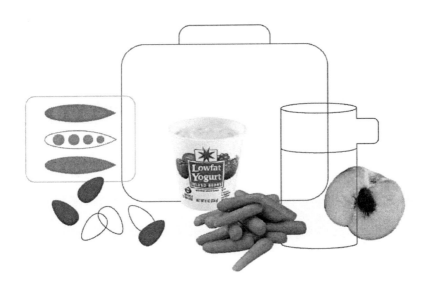

OVERVIEW

Many Americans consume more calories than they need without meeting recommended intakes for a number of nutrients. This circumstance means that most people need to choose meals and snacks that are high in nutrients but low to moderate in energy content; that is, meeting nutrient recommendations must go hand in hand with keeping calories under control. Doing so offers important benefits –normal growth and development of children, health promotion for people of all ages, and reduction of risk for a number of chronic diseases that are major public health problems.

Based on dietary intake data or evidence of public health problems, intake levels of the following nutrients may be of concern for:

- Adults: calcium, potassium, fiber, magnesium, and vitamins A (as carotenoids), C, and E,
- Children and adolescents: calcium, potassium, fiber, magnesium, and vitamin E,
- Specific population groups (see below): vitamin B_{12}, iron, folic acid, and vitamins E and D.

At the same time, in general, Americans consume too many calories and too much saturated and *trans* fats, cholesterol, added sugars, and salt.

DISCUSSION

Meeting Recommended Intakes Within Energy Needs

A basic premise of the *Dietary Guidelines* is that food guidance should recommend diets that will provide all the nutrients needed for growth and health. To this end, food guidance should encourage individuals to achieve the most recent nutrient intake recommendations of the Institute of Medicine, referred to collectively as the Dietary Reference Intakes (DRIs). Tables of the DRIs are provided at http://www.iom.edu/Object.File/Master/21/372/0.pdf.

An additional premise of the *Dietary Guidelines* is that the nutrients consumed should come primarily from foods. Foods contain not only the vitamins and minerals that are often found in supplements, but also hundreds of naturally occurring substances, including carotenoids, flavonoids and isoflavones, and protease inhibitors that may protect against chronic health conditions. There are instances when fortified foods may be advantageous, as identified in this chapter. These include providing additional sources of certain nutrients that might otherwise be present only in low amounts in some food sources, providing nutrients in highly bioavailable forms, and where the fortification addresses a documented public health need.

KEY RECOMMENDATIONS

- Consume a variety of nutrient-dense foods and beverages within and among the basic food groups while choosing foods that limit the intake of saturated and *trans* fats, cholesterol, added sugars, salt, and alcohol.
- Meet recommended intakes within energy needs by adopting a balanced eating pattern, such as the USDA Food Guide or the DASH Eating Plan.

Key Recommendations for Specific Population Groups

- *People over age 50.* Consume vitamin B_{12} in its crystalline form (i.e., fortified foods or supplements).
- *Women of childbearing age who may become pregnant.* Eat foods high in heme-iron and/or consume iron-rich plant foods or iron-fortified foods with an enhancer of iron absorption, such as vitamin C-rich foods.
- *Women of childbearing age who may become pregnant and those in the first trimester of pregnancy*
- Consume adequate synthetic folic acid daily (from fortified foods or supplements) in addition to food forms of folate from a varied diet.
- *Older adults, people with dark skin, and people exposed to insufficient ultraviolet band radiation (i.e., sunlight).* Consume extra vitamin D from vitamin D-fortified foods and/or supplements.

Two examples of eating patterns that exemplify the *Dietary Guidelines* are the DASH Eating Plan and the USDA Food Guide. These two similar eating patterns are designed to integrate dietary recommendations into a healthy way to eat and are used in the *Dietary Guidelines* to provide examples of how nutrient-focused recommendations can be expressed in terms of food choices. Both the USDA Food Guide and the DASH Eating Plan differ in important ways from common food consumption patterns in the United States. In general, they include:

- *More* dark green vegetables, orange vegetables, legumes, fruits, whole grains, and low-fat milk and milk products.
- *Less* refined grains, total fats (especially cholesterol, and saturated and *trans* fats), added sugars, and calories.

Both the USDA Food Guide and the DASH Eating Plan are constructed across a range of calorie levels to meet the nutrient needs of various age and gender groups. Table 1 provides food intake recommendations, and table 2 provides nutrient profiles for both the DASH Eating Plan and the USDA Food Guide at the 2,000-calorie level. These tables illustrate the many similarities between the two eating patterns. Additional calorie levels are shown in appendixes A-1 and A-2 for the USDA Food Guide and the DASH Eating Plan. The exact amounts of foods in these plans do not need to be achieved every day, but on average, over time. Table 3 can aid in identification of an individual's age, and physical activity level.

Variety Among and Within Food Groups

Each basic food group[1] is the major contributor of at least one nutrient while making substantial contributions of many other nutrients. Because each food group provides a wide array of nutrients in substantial amounts, it is important to include all food groups in the daily diet.

Both illustrative eating patterns include a variety of nutrient-dense foods within the major food groups. Selecting a variety of foods within the grain, vegetable, fruit, and meat groups may help to ensure that an adequate amount of nutrients and other potentially beneficial substances are consumed. For example, fish contains varying amounts of fatty acids that may be beneficial in reducing cardiovas-cular disease risk (see ch. 6).

Nutrient-Dense Foods

Nutrient-dense foods are those foods that provide substan -tial amounts of vitamins and minerals (micronutrients) and relatively few calories. Foods that are low in nutrient density are foods that supply calories but relatively small amounts of micronutrients, sometimes none at all. The greater the consumption of foods or beverages that are low in nutrient density, the more difficult it is to consume enough nutrients without gaining weight, especially for sedentary individuals. The consumption of added sugars, saturated and *trans* fats, and alcohol provides calories while providing little, if any, of the essential nutrients. (See ch. 7 for additional information on added sugars, ch. 6 for information on fats, and ch. 9 for information on alcohol.)

Selecting low-fat forms of foods in each group and forms free of added sugars – in other words nutrient-dense versions of foods – provides individuals a way to meet their nutrient needs while avoiding the overconsumption of calories and of food components such as saturated fats. However, Americans generally do not eat nutrient-dense forms of foods. Most people will exceed calorie recommendations if they consistently choose higher fat foods within the food groups – even if they do not have dessert, sweetened beverages, or alcoholic beverages.

If only nutrient-dense foods are selected from each food group in the amounts proposed, a small amount of calories can be consumed as added fats or sugars, alcohol, or other foods— *discretionary calorie allowance.* Appendixes A-2 and A-3 show the maximum discretionary calorie allowance that can be accommodated at each calorie level in the USDA Food Guide. Eating in accordance with the USDA Food Guide or the DASH Eating Plan will also keep intakes of saturated fat, total fat, and cholesterol within the limits recommended in chapter 6.

...meeting nutrient recommendations must go hand in hand with keeping calories under control.

Nutrients of Concern

The actual prevalence of inadequacy for a nutrient can be determined only if an Estimated Average Requirement (EAR) has been established and the distribution of usual dietary intake can be obtained. If such data are not avail- able for a nutrient but there is evidence for a public health problem associated with low intakes, in other words a nutrient might still -dense be considered to be of concern. provides individuals a way to meet

Based on these considerations, dietary intakes of the following nutrients may be low enough to be of concern for:

- Adults: calcium, potassium, fiber, magnesium, and vitamins A (as carotenoids), C, and E,
- Children and adolescents: even if they calcium, do not potassium, have dessert, fiber, magnesium, and vitamin E,
- Specific population groups: vitamin B_{12} · iron, folic acid, and vitamins E and D.

Efforts may be warranted to promote increased dietary intakes of potassium, fiber, and possibly vitamin E, regardless of age; increased intakes of calcium and possibly vitamins A (as carotenoids) and C and magnesium by adults; efforts are warranted to increase intakes of calcium and possibly magnesium by children age 9 years or older. Efforts may be especially warranted to improve the dietary intakes of adolescent females in general. Food sources of these nutrients are shown in appendix B.

Low intakes of fiber tend to reflect low intakes of whole grains, fruits, and vegetables. Low intakes of calcium tend to reflect low intakes of milk and milk products. Low intakes of vitamins A (as carotenoids) and C and magnesium tend to reflect low intakes of fruits and vegetables. Selecting fruits, vegetables, whole grains, and low-fat and fat-free milk and milk products in the amounts suggested by the USDA Food Guide and the DASH Eating Plan will provide adequate amounts of these nutrients.

Most Americans of all ages also need to increase their potassium intake. To meet the recommended potassium intake levels, potassium-rich foods from the fruit, vegetable, and dairy groups must be selected in both the USD A Food Guide and the DASH Eating Plan. Foods that can help increase potassium intake are listed in table 5 (ch. 5) and appendix B-1.

Most Americans may need to increase their consumption of foods rich in vitamin E (☐-tocopherol) while decreasing their intake of foods high in energy but low in nutrients. The vitamin E content in both the USDA Food Guide and the DASH Eating Plan is greater than current consumption, and specific vitamin E-rich foods need to be included in the eating patterns to meet the recommended intake of vitamin E. Foods that can help increase vitamin E intake are listed in appendix B-2, along with their calorie content. Breakfast cereal that is fortified with vitamin E is an option for individuals seeking to increase their vitamin E intake while consuming a low-fat diet.

In addition, most Americans need to decrease sodium intake. The DASH Eating Plan provides guidance on how to keep sodium intakes within recommendations. When using the USDA Food Guide, selecting foods that are lower in sodium than others is especially necessary to meet the recommended intake level at calorie levels of 2,600/day and above. Food choices that are lower in sodium are identi- fied in chapter 8.

Considerations for Specific Population Groups

People Over 50 and Vitamin B $_{12}$

Although a substantial proportion of individuals over age 50 have reduced ability to absorb naturally occurring vitamin B_{12}, they are able to absorb the crystalline form. Thus, all individuals over the age of 50 should be encour- aged to meet their Recommended Dietary Allowance (RDA) (2.4 $\square$g/day) for vitamin B_{12} by eating foods fortified with vitamin B_{12} such as fortified cereals, or by taking the crystalline form of vitamin B_{12} supplements.

Women and Iron

Based on blood values, substantial numbers of adolescent females and women of childbearing age are iron deficient. Thus, these groups should eat foods high in heme-iron (e.g., meats) and/or consume iron-rich plant foods (e.g., spinach) or iron-fortified foods with an enhancer of iron absorption, such as foods rich in vitamin C (e.g., orange juice). Appendix B-3 lists foods that can help increase iron intake and gives their iron and calorie content.

Women and Folic Acid

Since folic acid reduces the risk of the neural tube defects, spina bifida, and anencephaly, a daily intake of 400 µg/day of synthetic folic acid (from fortified foods or supplements in addition to food forms of folate from a varied diet) is recommended for women of childbearing age who may become pregnant. Pregnant women should consume 600 µg/day of synthetic folic acid (from fortified foods or supplements) in addition to food forms of folate from a varied diet. It is not known whether the same level of protection could be achieved by using food that is naturally rich in folate.

Special Groups and Vitamin D

Adequate vitamin D status, which depends on dietary intake and cutaneous synthesis, is important for optimal calcium absorption, and it can reduce the risk for bone loss. Two functionally relevant measures indicate that optimal serum 25-hydroxyvitamin D may be as high as 80 nmol/L. The elderly and individuals with dark skin (because the ability to synthesize vitamin D from exposure to sunlight varies with degree of skin pigmentation) are at a greater risk of low serum 25-hydroxyvitamin D concentrations. Also at risk are those exposed to insufficient ultraviolet radiation (i.e., sunlight) for the cutaneous production of vitamin D (e.g., housebound individuals). For individuals within the high-risk groups, substantially higher daily intakes of vitamin D (i.e., 25 □g or 1,000 International Units (IU) of vitamin D per day) have been recommended to reach and maintain serum 25-hydroxyvit- amin D values at 80 nmol/L. Three cups of vitamin D- fortified milk (7.5 □g or 300 IU), 1 cup of vitamin D-fortified orange juice (2.5 □g or 100 IU), and 15 □g (600 IU) of supplemental vitamin D would provide 25 □g (1,000 IU) of vitamin D daily.

Fluid

The combination of thirst and normal drinking behavior, especially the consumption of fluids with meals, is usually sufficient to maintain normal hydration. Healthy individuals who have routine access to fluids and who are not exposed to heat stress consume adequate water to meet their needs. Purposeful drinking is warranted for individuals who are exposed to heat stress or perform sustained vigorous activity (see ch. 4).

Flexibility of Food Patterns for Varied Food Preferences

The USDA Food Guide and the DASH Eating Plan are flexible to permit food choices based on individual and cultural food preferences, cost, and availability. Both can also accommodate varied types of cuisines and special needs due to common food allergies. Two adaptations of the USDA Food Guide and the DASH Eating Plan are:

Vegetarian Choices

Vegetarians of all types can achieve recommended nutrient intakes through careful selection of foods. These individuals should give special attention to their intakes of protein, iron, and vitamin B12, as well as calcium and vitamin D if avoiding milk products. In addition, vegetarians could select only nuts, seeds, and legumes from the meat and beans group, or they could include eggs if so desired. At the 2,000-calorie level, they could choose about 1.5 ounces of nuts and ²/₃ cup legumes instead of 5.5 ounces of meat, poultry, and/or fish. One egg, ½ ounce of nuts, or ¼ cup of legumes is considered equivalent to 1 ounce of meat, poultry, or fish in the USDA Food Guide. Substitutions for Milk and Milk Products

Since milk and milk products provide more than 70 percent of the calcium consumed by Americans, guidance on other choices of dietary calcium is needed for those who do not consume the recommended amount of milk products. Milk product consumption has been associated with overall diet quality and adequacy of intake of many nutrients, including calcium, potassium, magnesium, zinc, iron, riboflavin, vitamin A, folate, and vitamin D. People may avoid milk products because of allergies, cultural practices, taste, or other reasons. Those who avoid all milk products need to choose rich sources of the nutrients provided by milk, including potassium, vitamin A, and magnesium in addition to calcium and vitamin D (see app. B). Some non-dairy sources of calcium are shown in appendix B-4. The bioavailability of the calcium in these foods varies.

Those who avoid milk because of its lactose content may obtain all the nutrients provided by the milk group by using lactose-reduced or low-lactose milk products, taking small servings of milk several times a day, taking the enzyme lactase before consuming milk products, or eating other calcium-rich foods. For additional information, see appendixes B-4 and B-5 and NIH Publication No. 03-2751. [2]

Table 1. Sample USDA Food Guide and the DASH Eating Plan at the 2,000-Calorie Level [a]

Amounts of various food groups that are recommended each day or each week in the USDA Food Guide and in the DASH Eating Plan (amounts are daily unless otherwise specified) at the 2,000-calorie level. Also identified are equivalent amounts for different food choices in each group. To follow either eating pattern, food choices over time should provide these amounts of food from each group on average.

Food Groups and Subgroups	USDA Food Guide Amount[b]	DASH Eating Plan Amount	Equivalent Amounts
Fruit Group	2 cups (4 servings)	2 to 2.5 cups (4 to 5 servings)	$^1/_2$ cup equivalent is: • $^1/_2$ cup fresh, frozen, or canned fruit • 1 med fruit • $^1/_4$ cup dried fruit • USDA: $^1/_2$ cup fruit juice • DASH: $^3/_4$ cup fruit juice
Vegetable Group • Dark green vegetables • Orange vegetables • Legumes (dry beans) • Starchy vegetables • Other vegetables	2.5 cups (5 servings) 3 cups/week 2 cups/week 3 cups/week 3 cups/week 6.5 cups/week	2 to 2.5 cups (4 to 5 servings)	$^1/_2$ cup equivalent is: • $^1/_2$ cup of cut-up raw or cooked vegetable • 1 cup raw leafy vegetable • USDA: $^1/_2$ cup vegetable juice • DASH: $^3/_4$ cup vegetable juice
Grain Group • Whole grains • Other grains	6 ounce-equivalents 3 ounce-equivalents 3 ounce-equivalents	7 to 8 ounce-equivalents (7 to 8 servings)	1 ounce-equivalent is: • 1 slice bread • 1 cup dry cereal • $^1/_2$ cup cooked rice, pasta, cereal • DASH: 1 oz dry cereal ($^1/_{2}$ $_{1/4}$ cup depending on cereal type
Meat and Beans Group	5.5 ounce-equivalents	6 ounces or less meat, poultry, fish	1 ounce-equivalent is: • 1 ounce of cooked lean meats, poultry, fish

Table 1. Continued

Food Groups and Subgroups	USDA Food Guide Amount[b]	DASH Eating Plan Amount	Equivalent Amounts
Meat Beans Group (Continued)		4 to 5 servings per week nuts, seeds, and dry beans[c]	• 1 egg • USDA: ¼ cup cooked dry beans or tofu, 1 Tbsp peanut butter, ½ oz nuts or seeds • DASH: 1½ oz nuts, ½ oz seeds, ½ cup cooked dry beans
Milk Group	3 cups	2 to 3 cups	1 cup equivalent is: • 1 cup low-fat/fat-free milk, yogurt • 1½ oz of low-fat or fat-free natural cheese • 2 oz of low-fat or fat-free processed cheese
Oils	24 grams (6 tsp)	8 to 12 grams (2 to 3 tsp)	1 tsp equivalent is: • DASH: 1 tsp soft margarine • 1 Tbsp low-fat mayo • 2 Tbsp light salad dressing • 1 tsp vegetable oil
Discretionary Calorie Allowance • Example of distribution: Solid fat[d] Added sugars	267 calories 18 grams 8 tsp	 ~2 tsp (5 Tbsp per week)	1 Tbsp added sugar equivalent is: • DASH: 1 Tbsp jelly or jam • ½ oz jelly beans • 8 oz lemonade

[a] All servings are per day unless otherwise noted. USDA vegetable subgroup amounts and amounts of DASH nuts, seeds, and dry beans are per week.

[b] The 2,000-calorie USDA Food Guide is appropriate for many sedentary males 51 to 70 years of age, sedentary females 19 to 30 years of age, and for some other gender/age groups who are more physically active. See table 3 for information about gender/age/activity levels and appropriate calorie intakes. See appendixes A-2 and A-3 for more information on the food groups, amounts, and food intake patterns at other calorie levels.

[c] In the DASH Eating Plan, nuts, seeds, and dry beans are a separate food group from meat, poultry, and fish.

[d] The oils listed in this table are not considered to be part of discretionary calories because they are a major source of the vitamin E and polyunsaturated fatty acids, including the essential fatty acids, in the food pattern. In contrast, solid fats (i.e., saturated and *trans* fats) are listed separately as a source of discretionary calories.

Table 2. Comparison of Selected Nutrients in the Dietary Approaches to Stop Hypertension (DASH) Eating Plan[a], the USDA Food Guide[b], and Nutrient Intakes Recommended Per Day by the Institute of Medicine (IOM)[c]

Estimated nutrient levels in the DASH Eating Plan and the USDA Food Guide at the 2,000-calorie level, as well as the nutrient intake levels recommended by the Institute of Medicine for females 19—30 years of age.

Nutrient	DASH Eating Plan (2,000 kcals)	USDA Food Guide (2,000 kcals)	IOM Recommendations for Females 19 to 30
Protein, g	108	91	RDA: 46
Protein, % kcal	21	18	AMDR: 10
Carbohydrate, g	288	271	RDA: 130
Carbohydrate, % kcal	57	55	AMDR: 45
Total fat, g	48	65	
Total fat, % kcal	22	29	AMDR: 20
Saturated fat, g	10	17	
Saturated fat, % kcal	5	7.8	ALAP[d]
Monounsaturated fat, g	21	24	
Monounsaturated fat, % kcal	10	11	
Polyunsaturated fat, g	12	20	
Polyunsaturated fat, % kcal	5.5	9.0	
Linoleic acid, g	11	18	AI: 12
Alpha-linolenic acid, g	1	1.7	AI: 1.1
Cholesterol, mg	136	230	ALAP[d]
Total dietary fiber, g	30	31	AI: 28[e]
Potassium, mg	4,706	4,044	AI: 4,700
Sodium, mg	2,329[f]	1,779	AI: 1,500, UL: <2,300
Calcium, mg	1,619	1,316	AI: 1,000
Magnesium, mg	500	380	RDA: 310

Table 2. Continued

Nutrient	DASH Eating Plan	USDA Food Guide	IOM Recommendations
Copper, mg	2	1.5	RDA: 0.9
Iron, mg	21	18	RDA: 18
Phosphorus, mg	2,066	1,740	RDA: 700
Zinc, mg	14	14	RDA: 8
Thiamin, mg	2.0	2.0	RDA: 1.1
Riboflavin, mg	2.8	2.8	RDA: 1.1
Niacin equivalents, mg	31	22	RDA: 14
Vitamin B$_6$, mg	3.4	2.4	RDA: 1.3
Vitamin B$_{12}$, µg 7.1		8.3	RDA: 2.4
Vitamin C, mg	181	155	RDA: 75
Vitamin E (AT)[g]	16.5	9.5	RDA: 15.0
Vitamin A, µg (RAE)[h] 851		1,052	RDA: 700

[a] DASH nutrient values are based on a 1-week menu of the DASH Eating Plan. NIH publication No. 03-4082. www.nhlbi.nih.gov.

[b] USDA nutrient values are based on population-weighted averages of typical food choices within each food group or subgroup.

[c] Recommended intakes for adult females 19—30; DA = Recommended Dietary Allowance; AI = Adequate Intake; AMDR = Acceptable Macronutrient Distribution Range; UL = Upper Limit. R

[d] As Low As Possible while consuming a nutritionally adequate diet.

[e] Amount listed is based on 14 g dietary fiber/1,000 kcal.

[f] The DASH Eating Plan also can be used to follow at 1,500 mg sodium per day.

[g] AT = mg d-α-tocopherol

[h] RAE = Retinol Activity Equivalents

Table 3. Estimated Calorie Requirements (in Kilocalories) for Each Gender and Age Group at Three Levels of Physical Activity[a]

Estimated amounts of calories needed to maintain energy balance for various gender and age groups at three different levels of physical activity. The estimates are rounded to the nearest 200 calories and were determined using the Institute of Medicine equation.

| Gender | Age (years) | Activity Level[b,c,d] | | |
		Sedentary[b]	Moderately Active[c]	Active[d]
Child	2-3	1,000	1,000-1,400[e]	1,000-1,400[e]
Female	4-8	1,200	1,400-1,600	1,400-1,800
	9-13	1,600	1,600-2,000	1,800-2,200
	14-18	1,800	2,000	2,400
	19-30	2,000	2,000-2,200	2,400
	31-50	1,800	2,000	2,200
	50+	1,600	1,800	2,000-2,200
Male	4-8	1,400	1,400-1,600	1,600-2,000
	9-13	1,800	1,800-2,200	2,000-2,600
	14-18	2,200	2,400-2,800	2,800-3,200
	19-30	2,400	2,600-2,800	3,000
	31-50	2,200	2,400-2,600	2,800-3,000
	50+	2,000	2,200-2,400	2,400-2,800

[a] These levels are based on Estimated Energy Requirements (EER) from the Institute of Medicine Dietary Reference Intakes macronutrients report, 2002, calculated by gender, age, and activity level for reference-sized individuals. "Reference size," as BMI of 21.5 for adult females and 22.5 for adult males.

[b] Sedentary means a lifestyle that includes only the light physical activity associated with typical day-to-day life.

[c] Moderately active means a lifestyle that includes physical activity equivalent to walking about 1.5 to 3 miles per day at 3 to 4 miles per hour, in addition to the light physical activity associated with typical day-to-day life

[d] Active means a lifestyle that includes physical activity equivalent to walking more than 3 miles per day at 3 to 4 miles per hour, in addition to the light physical activity associated with typical day-to-day life.

[e] The calorie ranges shown are to accommodate needs of different ages within the group. For children and adolescents, more calories are needed at older ages. For adults, fewer calories are needed at older ages.

REFERENCES

[1] The food groups in the USDA Food Guide are grains; vegetables; fruits; milk, yogurt, and cheese; and meat, poultry, fish, dry beans, eggs, and nuts. Food groups in the DASH Eating Plan are grains and grain products; vegetables; fruits; low-fat or fat-free dairy; meat, poultry, and fish; and nuts, seeds, and dry beans.

[2] NIH Publication No. 03-2751, U.S. Department of Health and Human Services, National Institutes of Health, National Institute of Diabetes and Digestive and Kidney Diseases, March 2003. http://digestive. niddk.nih.gov/ddiseases/pubs/lactoseintolerance/index.htm.

In: Dietary Guide
Editor: Albert O. Gomber, pp. 35-43

ISBN: 1-59454-654-1
© 2007 Nova Science Publishers, Inc.

Chapter 3

WEIGHT MANAGEMENT

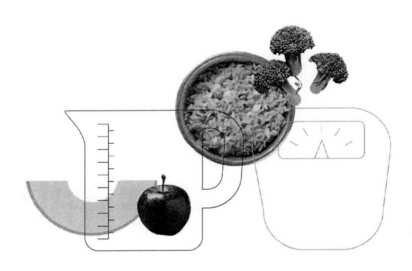

OVERVIEW

The prevalence of obesity in the United States has doubled in the past two decades. Nearly one-third of adults are obese, that is, they have a body mass index (BMI) of 30 or greater. One of the fastest growing segments of the population is that with a BM I$^>$ 30 with accompanying comorbidities. Over the last two decades, the prevalence of overweight among children and adolescents has increased substantially; it is estimated that as many as 16 percent of children and adolescents are overweight, representing a doubling of the rate among children and tripling of the rate among adolescents. A high prevalence of overweight and obesity is of great public health concern because excess body fat leads to a higher risk for premature death, type 2 diabetes, hypertension, dyslipidemia, cardiovascular disease, stroke, gall bladder disease, respiratory dysfunction, gout, osteoarthritis, and certain kinds of cancers.

Ideally, the goal for adults is to achieve and maintain a body weight that optimizes their health. However, for – obese adults, even modest weight loss (e.g., 10 pounds) has health benefits, and the prevention of further weight gain is very important. For overweight children and adolescents, the goal is to slow the rate of weight gain while achieving normal growth and development. Maintaining a healthy weight throughout childhood may reduce the risk of becoming an overweight or obese adult. Eating fewer calories while increasing physical activity are the keys to controlling body weight.

While overweight and obesity are currently significant public health issues, not all Americans need to lose weight. People at a healthy weight should strive to maintain their weight, and underweight individuals may need to increase their weight.

DISCUSSION

Overweight and obesity in the United States among adults and children has increased significantly over the last two decades. Those following typical American eating and activity patterns are likely to be consuming diets in excess of their energy requirements. However, caloric intake is only one side of the energy balance equation. Caloric expenditure needs to be in balance with caloric intake to maintain body weight and must exceed caloric intake to achieve weight loss (see tables 3 and 4). To reverse the trend toward obesity, most Americans need to eat fewer calories, be more active, and make wiser food choices.

Prevention of weight gain is critical because while the behaviors required are the same, the extent of the behaviors required to lose weight makes weight loss more challenging than prevention of weight gain. Since many adults gain weight slowly over time, even small decreases in calorie intake can help avoid weight gain, especially if accompanied by increased physical activity. For example, for most adults a reduction of 50 to 100 calories per day may prevent gradual weight gain, whereas a reduction of 500 calories or more per day is a common initial goal in weight-loss programs. Similarly, up to 60 minutes of moderate- to vigorous-intensity physical activity per day may be needed to prevent weight gain, but as much as 60 to 90 minutes of moderate-intensity physical activity per day is recommended to sustain weight loss for previously overweight people. It is advisable for men over age 40, women over age 50, and those with a history of chronic diseases such as heart disease or diabetes to consult with a healthcare provider before starting a vigorous exercise program. However, many people can safely increase their physical activity without consulting a healthcare provider. [1]

KEY RECOMMENDATIONS

- To maintain body weight in a healthy range, balance calories from foods and beverages with calories expended.
- To prevent gradual weight gain over time, make small decreases in food and beverage calories and increase physical activity.

Key Recommendations for Specific Population Groups

- *Those who need to lose weight.* Aim for a slow, steady weight loss by decreasing calorie intake while maintaining an adequate nutrient intake and increasing physical activity.
- *Overweight children.* Reduce the rate of body weight gain while allowing growth and development. Consult a healthcare provider before placing a child on a weight-reduction diet.
- *Pregnant women.* Ensure appropriate weight gain as specified by a healthcare provider.
- *Breastfeeding women.* Moderate weight reduction is safe and does not compromise weight gain of the nursing infant.
- *Overweight adults and overweight children with chronic diseases and/or on medication.* Consult a healthcare provider about weight loss strategies prior to starting a weight-reduction program to ensure appropriate management of other health conditions.

Monitoring body fat regularly can be a useful strategy for assessing the need to adjust caloric intake and energy expenditure. Two surrogate measures used to approximate body fat are BMI (adults and children) and waist circumference (adults).[2] BMI is defined as weight in kilograms divided by height, in meters, squared. For adults, weight status is based on the absolute BMI level (fig. 2). F or children and adolescents, weight status is determined by the comparison of the individual's BMI with age- and gender-specific percentile values (see fig. 3 for a sample boys' found at http://www.cdc.gov/growthcharts. BMI is more accurate at approximating body fat than is measuring body weight alone. However, BMI has some limitations. BMI overestimates body fat in people who are very muscular and underestimates body fat in people who have lost muscle mass. The relationship between BMI and body fat varies somewhat with age, gender, and ethnicity. In addition, for adults, BMI is a better predictor of a population's disease risk than an individual's risk of chronic disease.[8]

For children gaining excess weight, small decreases in energy intake reduce the rate at which they gain weight (body fat), thus improving their BMI percentile over time. As another surrogate measure, waist circumference can approximate abdominal fat but should be measured very carefully. Fat located in the abdominal region is associated with a greater health risk than peripheral fat. [8]

Some proposed calorie-lowering strategies include eating foods that are low in calories for a given measure of food (e.g., many kinds of vegetables and fruits and some soups). However, when making changes to improve nutrient intake, one needs to make substitutions to avoid excessive calorie intake. The healthiest way to reduce calorie intake is to reduce one's intake of added sugars, fats, and alcohol, which all provide calories but few or no essential nutrients (for more information, see chs. 6, 7, and 9).

Special attention should be given to portion sizes, which have increased significantly over the past two decades (http://hin.nhlbi.nih.gov/portion/index.htm). Though there are no empirical studies to show a causal relationship between increased portion sizes and obesity, there are studies showing that controlling portion sizes helps limit calorie intake, particularly when eating calorie-dense foods (foods that are high in calories for a given measure of food). Therefore, it is essential that the public understand how portion sizes compare to a recommended amount of food (i.e., serving) from each food group at a specific caloric level. The understanding of serving size and portion size is important in following either the DASH Eating Plan or the USDA Food Guide (see app. A). When using packaged foods with nutrient labels, people should pay attention to the units for serving sizes and how they compare to the serving sizes in the USDA Food Guide and the DASH Eating Plan.

Eating fewer calories while increasing physical activity are the keys to controlling body weight.

Lifestyle change in diet and physical activity is the best first choice for weight loss. A reduction in 500 calories or more per day is commonly needed. When it comes to intake of added sugars, body weight control, it is calories that count – not the proportions of fat, carbohydrates, and protein in the diet. However, when individuals are losing weight, they should follow a diet that is within the Acceptable Macronutrient Distribution Ranges (AMDR) for fat, carbohydrates, and protein, which are 20 to 35 percent of total calories, 45 to 65 percent of total calories, and 10 to 35 percent of total calories, respectively. Diets that provide very low or very high amounts of protein, carbohydrates, or fat are likely to provide low amounts of some nutrients and are not advisable for long-term use. Although these kinds of weight- loss diets have been shown to result in weight reduction, the maintenance of a reduced weight ultimately will depend on a change in lifestyle. Successful and sustainable weight loss and weight maintenance strategies require attention to both sides of the energy balance equation (i.e., caloric intake and energy expenditure).

Table 4. Calories/Hour Expended in Common Physical Activities

Some examples of physical activities commonly engaged in and the average amount of calories a 154-pound individual will expend by engaging in each activity for 1 hour. The expenditure value encompasses both resting metabolic rate calories and activity expenditure. Some of the activities can constitute either moderate- or vigorous-intensity physical activity depending on the rate at which they are carried out (for walking and bicycling).

Moderate Physical Activity	Approximate Calories/Hr for a 154 lb Person [a]
Hiking	370
Light gardening/yard work	330
Dancing	330
Golf (walking and carrying clubs)	330
Bicycling (<10 mph)	290
Walking (3.5 mph)	280
Weight lifting (general light workout)	220
Stretching	180
Vigorous Physical Activity	**Approximate Calories/Hr for a 154 lb Person [a]**
Running/jogging (5 mph)	590
Bicycling (>10 mph)	590
Swimming (slow freestyle laps)	510
Aerobics	480
Walking (4.5 mph)	460
Heavy yard work (chopping wood)	440
Weight lifting (vigorous effort)	440
Basketball (vigorous)	440

a Calories burned per hour will be higher for persons who weigh more than 154 lbs (70 kg) and lower for persons who weigh less.
Source: Adapted from the 2005 DGAC Report.

Figure 2 .Adult BMI Chart

Locate the height o f interest in the le ft-most column a nd read across the row for that height to the weight of interest. Follow t he colum n of the weigh t up to the top row th at lists the BMI . BMI of 18. 5—24 .9 is the healthy weight range, BMI of 25—29 .9 is the overweight range, and BMI o f 30 and above is in the obese range .

BMI	19	20	21	22	23	24	25	26	27	28	29	30	31	32	33	34	35
Height							Weight in Pounds										
4'10"	91	9 6	100	105	110	115	119	124	129	134	138	143	148	153	158	162	167
4'11"	94	99	104	109	114	119	124	12 8	133	138	143	148	153	158	163	168	173
5'	97	102	107	112	11 8	123	128	133	138	143	148	153	158	163	158	174	179
5'1"	100	10 6	111	11 6	122	127	132	137	143	148	153	158	164	169	174	180	185
5'2"	104	109	115	120	12 6	131	136	142	147	153	158	164	169	175	180	186	191
5'3"	107	113	11 8	124	130	135	141	146	152	158	163	169	175	180	186	191	197
5'4"	110	11 6	122	128	134	140	145	151	157	163	169	174	180	186	192	197	204
5'5"	114	120	12 6	132	138	144	150	156	162	168	174	180	186	192	198	204	210
5'6"	11 8	124	130	136	142	148	155	161	167	173	179	186	192	198	204	210	216
5'7"	121	127	134	140	14 6	153	159	166	172	178	185	191	198	204	211	217	223
5'8"	125	131	13 8	144	151	158	164	171	177	184	190	197	203	210	216	223	230
5'9"	12 8	135	142	149	155	162	169	176	182	189	196	203	209	216	223	230	236
5'10"	132	139	14 6	153	160	167	174	181	188	195	202	209	216	222	229	236	243
5'11"	13 6	143	150	157	1 65	172	179	186	193	200	208	215	222	229	236	243	250
6'	140	147	154	1 62	169	177	184	191	199	206	213	221	228	235	242	250	258
6'1"	144	151	159	1 66	174	182	189	197	204	212	219	227	235	242	250	257	265
6'2'	148	155	163	171	179	186	194	202	210	218	225	233	241	249	256	264	272
6'3'	152	1 60	168	176	184	192	200	208	216	224	232	240	248	256	264	272	279
	Healthy Weight						Overweight					Obese					

Source : Evidence Repor t o f Clinic a l G uidelines on t he Iden tification, Ev a l uation, and Tre ent o f Overweight and Obesity in Adu lts, 199 8. NIH/Nat ional Hea r t , L ung, and Blood Institute (NHLBI).

Calculate the BMI for an individual child using the following:
BMI = Weight (kg)/(Height [cm])^{2}x10,000 or BMI = Weight (lb)/(Height [in])^{2}x 703
Find the age of the child on the bottom, x-axis, and read up the chart from that age to the calculated BMI on the left and right, y-axis. The curve that is closest to the spot where the age and BMI of the child meet on the graph indicate the BMI percentile for this child relative to the population.

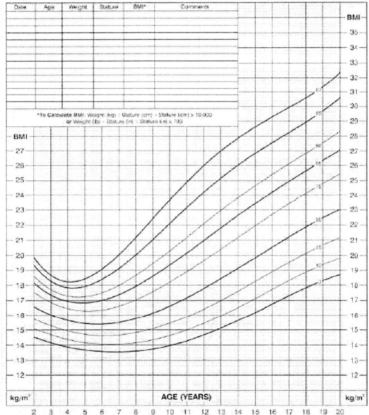

Figure 3. Example of Boys' BMI Growth Curve

Published May 30, 2000 (modified 10/16/00).
Source: Developed by the National Center for Health Statistics in collaboration with the National Center for Chronic Disease Pre vention and Health Promotion. http://www.cdc.gov/growthcharts (2000). Other growth charts are available at this source.

REFERENCES

[1] For more information on recommendations to consult a healthcare provider, see Physical Activity and Public Health—A vention and the Recommendation from American College of Sports Medicine, *JAMA* 273:402-407, 1995. http://wonder.cdc.gov/wonder/prevguid/p0000391/P0000391.asp.

[2] NIH Publication Number 00-4084, The Practical Guide: Identification, Evaluation and Treatment of Overweight and Obesity in Adults, U.S. Department of Health and Human Services, National Institutes of Health, National Heart, Lung, and Blood Institute, October 2000. http://www.nhlbi.nih.gov/guidelines/obesity/prctgd_c.pdf

In: Dietary Guide   ISBN: 1-59454-654-1
Editor: Albert O. Gomber, pp. 45-49   © 2007 Nova Science Publishers, Inc.

Chapter 4

PHYSICAL ACTIVITY

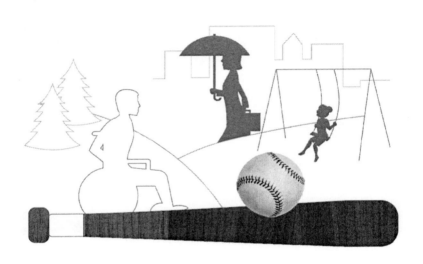

OVERVIEW

Americans tend to be relatively inactive. In 2002,25 percent of adult Americans did not participate in any leisure time physical activities in the past month,[1] and in 2003,38 percent of students in grades 9 to 12 viewed television3 or more hours per day.[2] Regular physical activity and physical fitness make important contributions to one's health, sense of well-being, and maintenance of a healthy body weight. Physical activity is defined as any bodily movement produced by skeletal muscles resulting in energy expenditure (http://www.cdc.gov/nccdphp/dnpa/physical/terms/index.htm).

In contrast, physical fitness is a multi-component trait related to the ability to perform physical activity. Maintenance of good physical fitness enables one to meet the physical demands of work and leisure comfortably. People with higher levels of physical fitness are also at lower risk of developing chronic disease. Conversely, a sedentary lifestyle increases risk for over weight and obesity and many chronic diseases, including coronary artery disease, hypertension, type 2 diabetes, osteoporosis, and certain types of cancer. Overall, mortality rates from all causes of death are lower in physically active people than in sedentary people. Also, physical activity can aid in managing mild to moderate depression and anxiety.

DISCUSSION

Regular physical activity has been shown to reduce the risk of certain chronic diseases, including high blood pressure, stroke, coronary artery disease, type 2 diabetes, colon cancer and osteoporosis. Therefore, to reduce the risk of chronic disease, it is recommended that adults engage in at least 30 minutes of moderate-intensity phys- ical activity on most, preferably all, days of the week. For most people, greater health benefits can be obtained by engaging in physical activity of more vigorous intensity or of longer duration. In addition, physical activity appears to promote psychological well-being and reduce feelings of mild to moderate depression and anxiety.

Regular physical activity is also a key factor in achieving and maintaining a healthy body weight for adults and children. To prevent the gradual accumulation of excess weight in adulthood, up to 30 additional minutes per day may be required over the 30 minutes for reduction of chronic disease risk and other health benefits. That is, approximately 60 minutes of moderate- to vigorous- intensity physical activity on most days of the week may be needed to prevent unhealthy weight gain (see table 4 for some examples of moderate- and vigorous-intensity physical activities). While moderate-intensity physical activity can achieve the desired goal, vigorous-intensity physical activity generally provides more benefits than moderate-intensity physical activity. Control of caloric intake is also advisable. However, to sustain weight loss for previously overweight/obese people, about 60 to 90 minutes of moderate-intensity physical activity per day is recommended.

KEY RECOMMENDATIONS

- Engage in regular physical activity and reduce sedentary activities to promote health, psychological well-being, and a healthy body weight.
- To reduce the risk of chronic disease in adulthood: Engage in at least 30 minutes of moderate-intensity physical activity, above usual activity, at work or home on most days of the week.
- For most people, greater health benefits can be obtained by engaging in physical activity of more vigorous intensity or longer duration.
- To help manage body weight and prevent gradual, unhealthy body weight gain in adulthood: Engage in approximately 60 minutes of moderate- to vigorous-intensity activity on most days of the week while not exceeding caloric intake requirements.
- To sustain weight loss in adulthood: Participate in at least 60 to 90 minutes of daily moderate-intensity physical activity while not exceeding caloric intake requirements. Some people may need to consult with a healthcare provider before participating in this level of activity.
- Achieve physical fitness by including cardiovascular conditioning, stretching exercises for flexibility, and resistance exercises or calisthenics for muscle strength and endurance.

Key Recommendations for Specific Population Groups

- *Children and adolescents.* Engage in at least 60 minutes of physical activity on most, preferably all, days of the week.
- *Pregnant women.* In the absence of medical or obstetric complications, incorporate 30 minutes or more of moderate-intensity physical activity on most, if not all, days of the week. Avoid activities with a high risk of falling or abdominal trauma.
- *Breastfeeding women.* Be aware that neither acute nor regular exercise adversely affects the to successfully breastfeed.
- *Older adults.* Participate in regular physical activity to reduce functional declines associated with aging and to achieve the other benefits of physical activity identified for all adults.

Most adults do not need to see their healthcare provider before starting a moderate-intensity physical activity program. However, men older than 40 years and women older than 50 years who plan a vigorous program or who have either chronic disease or risk factors for chronic disease should consult their physician to design a safe, effective program. It is also important during leisure time to limit sedentary behaviors, such as television watching and video viewing, and replace them with activities requiring more movement. Reducing these sedentary activities appears to be helpful in treating and preventing overweight among children and adolescents.

Different intensities and types of exercise confer different benefits. Vigorous physical activity (e.g., jogging or other aerobic exercise) provides greater benefits for physical fitness than does moderate physical activity and burns more calories per unit of time. Resistance exercise (such as weight training, using weight machines, and resistance band workouts) increases muscular strength and endurance and maintains or increases muscle mass. These benefits are seen in adolescents, adults, and older adults who perform resistance exercises on 2 or more days per week. Also, weight-bearing exercise has the potential to reduce the risk of osteoporosis by increasing peak bone mass during growth, maintaining peak bone mass during adult-hood, and reducing the rate of bone loss during aging. In addition, regular exercise can help prevent falls, which is of particular importance for older adults.

The barrier often given for a failure to be physically active is lack of time. Setting aside 30 to 60 consecutive minutes each day for planned exercise is one way to obtain physical activity, but it is not the only way. Physical activity may include short bouts (e.g., 10-minute bouts) of moderate-intensity activity. The accumulated total is what is important – both for health and for burning calories. Physical activity can be accumulated through three to six 10-minute bouts over the course of a day.

Elevating the level of daily physical activity may also provide indirect nutritional benefits. A sedentary lifestyle limits the number of calories that can be consumed without gaining weight. The higher a person's physical activity level, the higher his or her energy requirement and the easier it is to plan a daily food intake pattern that meets recommended nutrient requirements.

Proper hydration is important when participating in phys-ical activity. Two steps that help avoid dehydration during prolonged physical activity or when it is hot include: (1) consuming fluid regularly during the activity and (2) drinking several glasses of water or other fluid after the physical activity is completed (see chs. 2 and 8).

Regular physical activity and physical fitness make important contri-butions to one's health, sense of well-being, and maintenance of a healthy body weight.

REFERENCES

[1]   Behavioral Risk Factor Surveillance System, Surveillance for Certain Health Behaviors Among Selected Local Areas—United States, Behavioral Risk Factor Surveillance System, 2002, *Morbidity and Mortality Weekly Report (MMWR)*, **53**, No SS-05. http://www.cdc.gov/brfss/.

[2]   Youth Risk Behavior Surveillance System, Youth Risk Behavior Surveillance—United States, 2003 *MMWR* **53**(SS-2):1–29, 2004. http://www.cdc.gov/healthyyouth/yrbs/.

In: Dietary Guide   ISBN: 1-59454-654-1
Editor: Albert O. Gomber, pp. 51-58   © 2007 Nova Science Publishers, Inc.

Chapter 5

FOOD GROUPS TO ENCOURAGE

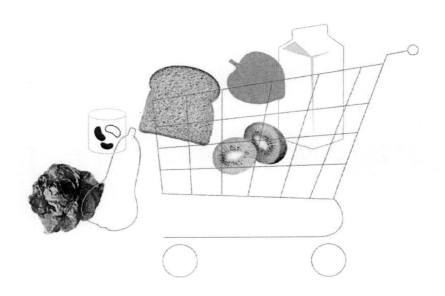

OVERVIEW

Increased intakes of fruits, vegetables, whole grains, and fat-free or low-fat milk and milk products are likely to have important health benefits for most Americans. While protein is an important macronutrient in the diet, most Americans are already currently consuming enough (AMDR = 10 to 35 percent of calories) and do not need to increase their intake. As such, protein consumption, while important for nutrient adequacy, is not a focus of this document. Although associations have been identified between specific food groups (e.g., fruits and vegetables) and reduced risk for chronic diseases, the effects are inter-related and the health benefits should be considered in the context of an overall healthy diet that does not exceed calorie needs (such as the USDA Food Guide or the DASH Eating Plan; see ch. 2). The strength of the evidence for the association between increased intake of fruits and vegetables and reduced risk of chronic diseases is variable and depends on the specific disease, but an array of evidence points to beneficial health effects.

Compared with the many people who consume a dietary pattern with only small amounts of fruits and vegetables, those who eat more generous amounts as part of a healthful diet are likely to have reduced risk of chronic diseases, including stroke and perhaps other cardiovascular diseases, type 2 diabetes, and cancers in certain sites (oral cavity and pharynx, larynx, lung, esophagus, stomach, and colon-rectum). Diets rich in foods containing fiber, such as fruits, vegetables, and whole grains, may reduce the risk of coronary heart disease. Diets rich in milk and milk products can reduce the risk of low bone mass throughout the life cycle. The consumption of milk products is especially important for children and adolescents who are building their peak bone mass and developing lifelong habits. Although each of these food groups may have a different relationship with disease outcomes, the adequate consumption of all food groups contributes to overall health.

DISCUSSION

Fruits, vegetables, whole grains, and milk products are all important to a healthful diet and can be good sources of the nutrients of concern (see ch. 2). When increasing intake of fruits, vegetables, whole grains, and fat-free or low-fat milk and milk products, it is important to decrease one's intake of less-nutrient-dense foods to control calorie intake. The 2,000-calorie level used in the discussion is a reference level only; it is not a recommended calorie intake because many Americans should be consuming fewer calories to maintain a healthy weight.

Fruits and Vegetables

Four and one-half cups (nine servings) of fruits and vegetables are recommended daily for the reference 2,000-calorie level, with higher or lower amounts depending on the caloric level. This results in a range of 2 ½ to 6½ cups (5 to 13 servings) of fruits and vegetables each day for the 1,200- to 3,200-calorie levels [1] (app. A-2). Fruits and vegetables provide a variety of micronutrients and fiber. Table 5 provides a list of fruits and vegetables that are good sources of vitamins A (as carotenoids) and C, folate, and potassium.

KEY RECOMMENDATIONS

- Consume a sufficient amount of fruits and vegetables while staying within energy needs. Two cups of fruit and $2^1/_2$ cups of vegetables per day are recommended for a reference 2,000-calorie intake, with higher or lower amounts depending on the calorie level.
- Choose a variety of fruits and vegetables each day. In particular, select from all five vegetable subgroups (dark green, orange, legumes, starchy vegetables, and other vegetables) several times a week.
- Consume 3 or more ounce-equivalents of whole-grain products per day, with the rest of the recommended grains coming from enriched or whole-grain products. In general, at least half the grains should come from whole grains.
- Consume 3 cups per day of fat-free or low-fat milk or equivalent milk products.

Key Recommendations for Specific Population Groups

- *Children and adolescents.* Consume whole-grain products often; at least half the grains should be whole grains. Children 2 to 8 years should consume 2 cups per day of fat-free or low-fat milk or equivalent milk products. Children 9 years of age and older should consume 3 cups per day of fat-free or low-fat milk or equivalent milk products.

In the fruit group, consumption of whole fruits (fresh, frozen, canned, dried) rather than fruit juice for the majority of the total daily amount is suggested to ensure adequate fiber intake. Different vegetables are rich in different nutrients. In the vegetable group, weekly intake of specific amounts from each of five vegetable subgroups (dark green, orange, legumes [dry beans], starchy, and other vegetables)[2] is recommended for adequate nutrient intake. Each subgroup provides a some-what different array of nutrients. In the USDA Food Guide at the reference 2,000-calorie level, the following weekly amounts are recommended:

Dark green vegetables	3 cups/week
Orange vegetables	2 cups/week
Legumes (dry beans)	3 cups/week
Starchy vegetables	3 cups/week
Other vegetables	$6\frac{1}{2}$ cups/week

Most current consumption patterns do not achieve the recommended intakes of many of these vegetables. The DASH Eating Plan and the USDA Food Guide suggest increasing intakes of dark green vegetables, orange vegetables, and legumes (dry beans) as part of the overall recommendation to have an adequate intake of fruits and vegetables (see ch. 2).

Whole Grains

In addition to fruits and vegetables, whole grains are an important source of fiber and other nutrients. Whole grains, as well as foods made from them, consist of the entire grain seed, usually called the kernel. The kernel is made of three components – the bran, the germ, and the endosperm. If the kernel has been cracked, crushed, or flaked, then it must retain nearly the same relative proportions of bran, germ, and endosperm as the original grain to be called whole grain. In the grain-refining process, most of the bran and some of the germ is removed, resulting in the loss of dietary fiber (also known as cereal fiber), vitamins, minerals, lignans, phytoestrogens, phenolic compounds, and phytic acid. Some manufacturers add bran to grain products to increase the dietary fiber content. Refined grains are the resulting product of the grain-refining processing. Most refined grains are enriched before being further processed into foods. Enriched refined grain products that conform to standards of identity are required by law to be fortified with folic acid, as well as thiamin, riboflavin, niacin, and iron. Food manufacturers may fortify whole-grain foods where regulations permit the addition of folic acid. Currently, a number of whole-grain, ready-to-eat breakfast cereals are fortified with folic acid. As illustrated by the comparison of whole-wheat and enriched white flours in table 6, many nutrients occur at higher or similar levels in whole grains when compared to enriched grains, but whole grains have less folate unless they have been fortified with folic acid.

Consuming at least 3 or more ounce-equivalents of whole grains per day can reduce the risk of several chronic diseases and may help with weight maintenance. Thus, daily intake of at least 3 ounce-equivalents of whole grains per day is recommended by substituting whole grains for refined grains. However, because three servings may be difficult for younger children to achieve, it is recommended that they increase whole grains into their diets as they grow. At all calorie levels, all age groups should consume at least half the grains as whole grains to achieve the fiber recommendation. All grain servings can be whole-grain; however, it is advisable to include some folate-fortified products, such as folate-fortified whole-grain cereals, in these whole-grain choices.

Increased intakes of fruits, vegetables, whole grains, and fat-free or low-fat milk and milk products are likely to have important health benefits for most Americans.

Whole grains cannot be identified by the color of the food; label-reading skills are needed. Table 7 identifies names of whole grains that are available in the United States. For information about the ingredients in whole-grain and enriched-grain products, read the ingredient list on the food label. For many whole-grain products, the words "whole" or "whole grain will appear before the grain ingredient's name. The whole grain should be the first ingredient listed. Wheat flour, enriched flour, and degerminated cornmeal are not whole grains. The Food and Drug Administration requires foods that bear the whole-grain health claim to (1) contain 51 percent or more whole-grain ingredients by weight per reference amount and (2) be low in fat.

Milk and Milk Products

Another source of nutrients is milk and milk products. Milk product consumption has been associated with overall diet quality and adequacy of intake of many nutri-ents. The intake of milk products is especially important to bone health during childhood and adolescence. Studies specifically on milk and other milk products, such as yogurt and cheese, showed a positive relationship between the intake of milk and milk products and bone mineral content or bone mineral density in one or more skeletal sites (see table 1 for information on equivalent amounts of milk products).

Adults and children should not avoid milk and milk prod- ucts because of concerns that these foods lead to weight gain. There are many fat-free and low-fat choices without added sugars that are available and consistent with an overall healthy dietary plan. If a person wants to consider milk alternatives because of lactose intolerance, the most reliable and easiest ways to derive the health benefits associated with milk and milk product consumption is to choose alternatives within the milk food group, such as yogurt or lactose-free milk, or to consume the enzyme lactase prior to the consumption of milk products. For individuals who choose to or must avoid all milk products (e.g., individuals with lactose intolerance, vegans), non-dairy calcium-containing alternatives may be selected to help meet calcium needs (app. B-4).

Table 5. Fruits, Vegetables, and Legumes (Dry Beans) That Contain Vitamin A (Carotenoids), Vitamin C, Folate, and Potassium

Many of the fruits, vegetables, and legumes (beans) are considered to be important sources of vitamin A (as carotenoids), vitamin C, and potassium in the adult population. Intakes of these nutrients, based on dietary intake data or evidence of public health problems, may be of concern. Also listed are sources of naturally occurring folate, a nutrient considered to be of concern for women of childbearing age and those in the first trimester of pregnanc y. Folic acid- fortified grain products, not listed in this table, are also good sources.

Sources of vitamin A (carotenoids) (see app. B-6)
• Bright orange vegetables like carrots, sweetpotatoes, and pumpkin
• Tomatoes and tomato products, red sweet pepper
• Leafy greens such as spinach, collards, turnip greens, kale, beet and mustard greens, green leaf lettuce, and romaine
• Orange fruits like mango, cantaloupe, apricots, and red or pink grapefruit

Sources of vitamin C
• Citrus fruits and juices, kiwi fruit, strawberries, guava, papaya, and cantaloupe
• Broccoli, peppers, tomatoes, cabbage (especially Chinese cabbage), brussels sprouts, and potatoes
• Leafy greens such as romaine, turnip greens, and spinach

Sources of folate
• Cooked dry beans and peas
• Oranges and orange juice
• Deep green leaves like spinach and mustard greens

Sources of potassium (see app. B-1)
• Baked white or sweetpotatoes, cooked greens (such as spinach), winter (orange) squash
• Bananas, plantains, many dried fruits, oranges and orange juice, cantaloupe, and honeydew melons
• Cooked dry beans
• Soybeans (green and mature)
• Tomato products (sauce, paste, puree)
• Beet greens

Table 6. Comparison of 100 Grams of Whole-Grain Wheat Flour and Enriched, Bleached, White, All-Purpose Flour

Some of the nutrients of concern and the fortification nutrients in 100 percent whole-wheat flour and enriched, bleached, all-purpose white (wheat) flour. Dietary fiber, calcium, magnesium and potassium, nutrients of concern, occur in much higher concentrations in the whole-wheat flour on a 100-gram basis (percent). The fortification nutrients—thiamin, riboflavin, niacin, and iron –are similar in concentration between the two flours, but folate, as Dietar y Folate Equivalent (DFE), µg, is higher in the enriched white flour.

	100 Percent Whole-Grain Wheat Flour	Enriched, Bleached, All-Purpose White Flour
Calories, kcal	339.0	364.0
Dietary fiber, g	12.2	2.7
Calcium, mg	34.0	15.0
Magnesium, mg	138.0	22.0
Potassium, mg	405.0	107.0
Folate, DFE, µg	44.0	291.0
Thiamin, mg	0.5	0.8
Riboflavin, mg	0.2	0.5
Niacin, mg	6.4	5.9
Iron, mg	3.9	4.6

Source: Agricultural Research Service Nutrient Database for Standard Reference, Release 17.

Table 7. Whole Grains Available in the United States

Whole grains that are consumed in the United States either as a single food (e.g., wild rice, popcorn) or as an ingredient in a multi-ingredient food (e.g., in multi-grain breads). This listing of whole grains was determined from a breakdown of foods reported consumed in nationwide food consumption surveys, by amount consumed. The foods are listed in approximate order of amount consumed, but the order may change over time. In addition, other whole grains may be consumed that are not yet represented in the surveys.

Whole wheat
Whole oats/oatmeal
Whole-grain corn
Popcorn
Brown rice
Whole rye
Whole-grain barley
Wild rice
Buckwheat
Triticale
Bulgur (cracked wheat)
Millet
Quinoa
Sorghum

Source: Agriculture Research Service Database for C SFII 1994

REFERENCES

[1] See appendix A-2 and table D1-16 from the 2005 DG AC Report (or USDA website) for information on children age 2 to 3 years.

[2] Includes all fresh, frozen, canned, cooked, or raw forms of vegetables. Examples of vegetables are dark green (broccoli, spinach, most greens); orange (carrots, sweetpotatoes, winter squash, pumpkin); legumes (dry beans, chickpeas, tofu); starchy (corn, white potatoes, green peas); other (tomatoes, cabbage, celery, cucumber, lettuce, onions, peppers, green beans, cauliflower, mush-rooms, summer squash).

In: Dietary Guide   ISBN: 1-59454-654-1
Editor: Albert O. Gomber, pp. 59-67 © 2007 Nova Science Publishers, Inc.

Chapter 6

FATS

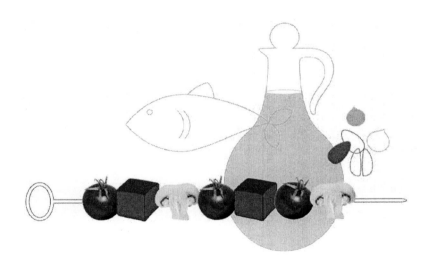

OVERVIEW

Fats and oils are part of a healthful diet, but the type of fat makes a difference to heart health, and the total amount of fat consumed is also important. High intake of saturated fats, *trans* fats, and cholesterol increases the risk of unhealthy blood lipid levels, which, in turn, may increase the risk of coronary heart disease. A high intake of fat (greater than 35 percent of calories) generally increases saturated fat intake and makes it more difficult to avoid consuming excess calories. A low intake of fats and oils (less than 20 percent of calories) increases the risk of inad- equate intakes of vitamin E and of essential fatty acids and may contribute to unfavorable changes in high-density lipoprotein (HDL) blood cholesterol and triglycerides.

DISCUSSION

Fats supply energy and essential fatty acids and serve as a carrier for the absorption of the fat-soluble vitamins A,D, E,and K and carotenoids. Fats serve as building blocks of membranes and play a key regulatory role in numerous biological functions. Dietary fat is found in foods derived from both plants and animals. The recommended total fat intake is between 20 and 35 percent of calories for adults. A fat intake of 30 to 35 percent of calories is recommended for children 2 to 3 years of age and 25 to 35 percent of calories for children and adolescents 4 to 18 years of age. Few Americans consume less than 20 percent of calories from fat. Fat intakes that exceed 35 percent of calories are associated with both total increased saturated fat and calorie intakes.

To decrease their risk of elevated low-density lipoprotein (LDL) cholesterol in the blood, most Americans need to decrease their intakes of saturated fat and *trans* fats, and many need to decrease their dietary intake of cholesterol. Because men tend to have higher intakes of dietary cholesterol, it is especially important for them to meet this recommendation. Population-based studies of American diets show that intake of saturated fat is more excessive than intake of *trans* fats and cholesterol. Therefore, it is most important for Americans to decrease their intake of saturated fat. However, intake of all three should be decreased to meet recommendations. Table 8 shows, for selected calorie levels, the maximum gram amounts of saturated fat to consume to keep saturated fat intake below 10 percent of total calorie intake. This table may be useful when combined with label-reading guidance. Table 9 gives a few practical examples of the differences in the saturated fat content of different forms of commonly consumed foods. Table 10 provides the major dietary sources of saturated fats in the U.S. diet listed in decreasing order. Diets can be planned to meet nutrient recommendations for linoleic acid and α-linolenic acid while providing very low amounts of saturated fatty acids.

Based on 1994-1996 data, the estimated average daily intake of *trans* fats in the United States was about 2.6 percent of total energy intake. Processed foods and oils provide approximately 80 percent of *trans* fats in the diet, compared to 20 percent that occur naturally in food from animal sources. Table 11 provides the major dietary sources of *trans* fats listed in decreasing order. *Trans* fat content of certain processed foods has changed and is likely to continue to change as the industry reformulates products. Because the *trans* fatty acids produced in the partial hydrogenation of vegetable oils account for more than 80 percent of total intake, the food industry has an important role in decreasing *trans* fatty acid content of the food supply. Limited consumption of foods made with processed sources of *trans* fats provides the most effective means of reducing intake of *trans* fats. By looking at the food label, consumers can select products that are lowest in saturated fat, *trans* fats,[1] and cholesterol.

KEY RECOMMENDATIONS

- Consume less than 10 percent of calories from saturated fatty acids and less than 300 mg/day of cholesterol, and keep *trans* fatty acid consumption as low as possible.
- Keep total fat intake between 20 to 35 percent of calories, with most fats coming from sources of polyunsaturated and monounsaturated fatty acids, such as fish, nuts, and vegetable oils.
- When selecting and preparing meat, poultry, dry beans, and milk or milk products, make choices that are lean, low-fat, or fat-free.
- Limit intake of fats and oils high in saturated and/or *trans* fatty acids, and choose products low in such fats and oils.

Key Recommendations for Specific Population Groups

- *Children and adolescents.* Keep total fat intakebetween 30 to 35 percent of calories for children 2 to 3 years of age and between 25 to 35 percent of calo - ries for children and adolescents 4 to 18 years of age , with most fats coming from sources of polyunsatu- rated and monounsaturated fatty acids, such as fish, nuts, and vegetable oils.

To meet the total fat recommendation of 20 to 35 percent of calories, most dietary fats should come from sources of polyunsaturated and monounsaturated fatty acids. Sources of omega-6 polyunsaturated fatty acids are liquid vegetable oils, including soybean oil, corn oil, and safflower oil. Plant sources of omega-3 polyunsaturated fatty acids (α-linolenic acid) include soybean oil, canola oil, walnuts, and flaxseed. Eicosapentaenoic acid (EPA) and docosahexaenoic acid (DHA) are omega-3 fatty acids that are contained in fish and shellfish. Fish that naturally contain more oil (e.g., salmon, trout, herring) are higher in EPA and DHA than are lean fish (e.g., cod, haddock, catfish). Limited evidence suggests an association between consumption of fatty acids in fish and reduced risks of mortality from cardiovascular disease for the general population. Other sources of EPA and DHA may provide similar benefits; however, more research is needed. Plant sources that are rich in monounsaturated fatty acids include vegetable oils (e.g., canola, olive, high oleic safflower, and sunflower oils) that are liquid at room temperature and nuts.

Considerations for Specific Population Groups

Evidence suggests that consuming approximately two servings of fish per week (approximately 8 ounces total) may reduce the risk of mortality from coronary heart disease and that consuming EPA and DHA may reduce the risk of mortality from cardiovascular disease in people who have already experienced a cardiac event.

Federal and State advisories provide current information about lowering exposure to environmental contaminants in fish. For example, methylmercury is a heavy metal toxin found in varying levels in nearly all fish and shellfish. F or most people, the risk from mercury by eating fish and shellfish is not a health concern. However, some fish contain higher levels of mercury that may harm an unborn baby or young child's developing nervous system. The risks from mercury in fish and shellfish depend on the amount of fish eaten and the levels of mercury in the fish. Therefore, the Food and Drug Administration (FDA) and the Environmental Protection Agency are advising women of childbearing age who may become pregnant, pregnant women, nursing mothers, and young children to avoid some types of fish and shellfish and eat fish and shellfish food information line toll-free at 1-888-SAFEFOOD or visit http://www.cfsan.fda.gov/~dms/admehg3.html.

...most Americans need to decrease their intakes of saturated fat and trans fats, and many need to decrease their dietary intake of cholesterol.

Lower intakes (less than 7 percent of calories from satu- rated fat and less than 200 mg/day of cholesterol) are recommended as part of a therapeutic diet for adults with elevated LDL blood cholesterol (i.e., above their LDL blood FDA's cholesterol goal [see table 12]). People with an elevated LDL blood cholesterol level should be under the care of a healthcare provider.

Table 8. Maximum Daily Amounts of Saturated Fat To Keep Saturated Fat Below 10 Percent of Total Calorie Intake

The maximum gram amounts of saturated fat that can be consumed to keep saturated fat intake below 10 percent of total calorie intake for selected calorie levels. A 2,000-calorie example is included for consistency with the food label. This table may be useful when combined with label- reading guidance.

Total Calorie Intake	Limit on Saturated Fat Intake
1,600	18 g or less
2,000[a]	20 g or less
2,200	24 g or less
2,500[a]	25 g or less
2,800	31 g or less

[a] Percent Daily Values on the Nutrition Facts Panel of food labels are based on a 2,000-calorie diet. Values for 2,000 and 2,500 calories are rounded to the nearest 5 grams to be consistent with the Nutrition Facts Panel.

Table 9. Differences in Saturated Fat and Calorie Content of Commonly Consumed Foods

This table shows a few practical examples of the differences in the saturated fat content of different forms of commonly consumed foods. Comparisons are made between foods in the same food group (e.g., regular cheddar cheese and low-fat cheddar cheese), illustrating that lower saturated fat choices can be made within the same food group.

Food Category	Portion	Saturated Fat Content (grams)	Calories
Cheese			
• Regular cheddar cheese	1 oz	6.0	114
• Low-fat cheddar cheese	1 oz	1.2	49
Ground beef			
• Regular ground beef (25% fat)	3 oz (cooked)	6.1	236
• Extra lean ground beef (5% fat)	3 oz (cooked)	2.6	148
Milk			
• Whole milk (3.24%)	1 cup	4.6	146
• Low-fat (1%) milk	1 cup	1.5	102
Breads			
• Croissant (med)	1 medium	6.6	231
• Bagel, oat bran (4")	1 medium	0.2	227
Frozen desserts			
• Regular ice cream	$^1/_2$ cup	4.9	145
• Frozen yogurt, low-fat	$^1/_2$ cup	2.0	110
Table spreads			
• Butter	1 tsp	2.4	34
• Soft margarine with zero *trans*	1 tsp	0.7	25
Chicken			
• Fried chicken (leg with skin)	3 oz (cooked)	3.3	212
• Roasted chicken (breast no skin)	3 oz (cooked)	0.9	140
Fish			
• Fried fish	3 oz	2.8	195
• Baked fish	3 oz	1.5	129

Source: ARS Nutrient Database for Standard Reference, Release 17.

Table 10. Contribution of Various Foods to Saturated Fat Intake in the American Diet (Mean Intake = 25.5 g)

The major dietary sources of saturated fats in the U.S. diet listed in decreasing order.

Food Group	Contribution (percent of total sat fat consumed)
Cheese	13.1
Beef	11.7
Milk[a]	7.8
Oils	4.9
Ice cream/sherbet/frozen yogurt	4.7
Cakes/cookies/quick breads/doughnuts	4.7
Butter	4.6
Other fats[b]	4.4
Salad dressings/mayonnaise	3.7
Poultry	3.6
Margarine	3.2
Sausage	3.1
Potato chips/corn chips/popcorn	2.9
Yeast bread	2.6
Eggs	2.3

[a] The milk category includes all milk, including whole milk, low-fat milk, and fat-free milk.
[b] Shortening and animal fats
Source: Adapted from Cotton PA, Subar AF, Friday JE, Cook A, Dietary Sources of Nutrients among U.S. Adults, 1994–1996. *JADA* 104:921-931, 2004.

**Table 11. Contribution of Various Foods to *Trans* Fat Intake in the
American Diet (Mean Intake = 5.84 g)**

The major dietary sources of *trans* fats listed in decreasing order. Processed foods and oils provide approximately 80 percent of *trans* fats in the diet, compared to 20 percent that occur naturally in food from animal sources. *Trans* ats content of certain processed foods has changed and is likely to continue to change as the industry reformulates products.

Food Group	Contribution (percent of total *trans* fats consumed)
Cakes, cookies, crackers, pies, bread, etc.	40
Animal products	21
Margarine	17
Fried potatoes	8
Potato chips, corn chips, popcorn	5
Household shortening	4
Other[a]	5

[a] Includes breakfast cereal and candy. USDA analysis reported 0 grams of *trans* fats in salad dressing.

Source: Adapted from *Federal Register* notice. *Food Labeling; Trans Fatty Acids in Nutrition Labeling; Consumer Research To Consider Nutrient Content and Health Claims and Possible Footnote or Disclosure Statements; Final Rule and Proposed Rule* . Vol. 68, No. 133, p. 41433-41506, July 11, 2003. Data collected 1994-1996.

Table 12. Relationship Between LDL Blood Cholesterol Goal and the Level of Coronar y Heart Disease Risk

Information for adults with elevated LD L blood cholesterol. LDL blood cholesterol goals for these individuals are related to the level of coronary heart disease risk. People with an elevated LDL blood cholesterol value should make therapeutic lifestyle changes (diet, physical activity, weight control) under the care of a healthcare provider to lower LDL blood cholesterol.

If Someone Has:	LDL Blood Cholesterol Goal Is:
CHD or CHD risk equivalent[a]	Less than 100 mg/dL
Two or more risk factors other than elevated LDL blood cholesterol [b]	Less than 130 mg/dL
Zero or one risk factor other than elevated LDL blood cholesterol [b]	Less than 160 mg/dL

[a] CHD (coronary heart disease) risk equivalent = presence of clinical atherosclerotic disease that
    confers high risk for CHD events:
    -Clinical CHD
    -Symptomatic carotid artery disease
    -Peripheral arterial disease
    -Abdominal aortic aneurysm
    -Diabetes
    -Two or more risk factors with >20% risk for CH D (or myocardial infarction or CHD
        death) within 10 years
b Major risk factors that affect your LDL goal:
    -Cigarette smoking
    -High blood pressure (140/90 mmHg or higher or on blood pressure medication)
    - Low HDL blood cholesterol (less than 40 mg/dL)
    -Family history of early heart disease (heart disease in father or brother before age 55;
        heart disease in mother or sister before age 65)
    -Age (men 45 years or older; women 55 years or older)
Source: NIH Publication No. 01-3290, U.S. Department of Health and Human Services, National Institutes of Health, National Heart, Lung, and Blood Institute, National Cholesterol Education Program Brochure, High Blood Cholesterol What You Need to Know, May 2001. http://www.nhlbi.nih.gov/health/public/heart/chol/hbc_what.htm.

REFERENCES

[1]   Including the amount of *trans* fats on the Nutrition Facts Panel is voluntary until January 2006.

In: Dietary Guide   ISBN: 1-59454-654-1
Editor: Albert O. Gomber, pp. 69-75 © 2007 Nova Science Publishers, Inc.

Chapter 7

CARBOHYDRATES

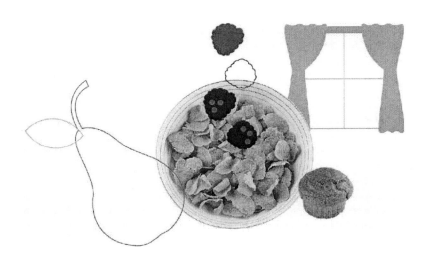

OVERVIEW

Carbohydrates are part of a healthful diet. The AMDR for carbohydrates is 45 to 65 percent of total calories. Dietary fiber is composed of nondigestible carbohydrates and lignin intrinsic and intact in plants. Diets rich in dietary fiber have been shown to have a number of beneficial effects, including decreased risk of coronary heart disease and improvement in laxation. There is also interest in the potential relationship between diets containing fiber-rich foods and lower risk of type 2 diabetes. Sugars and starches supply energy to the body in the form of glucose, which is the only energy source for red blood cells and is the preferred energy source for the brain, central nervous system, placenta, and fetus. Sugars can be naturally present in foods (such as the fructose in fruit or the lactose in milk) or added to the food. Added sugars, also known as caloric sweeteners, are sugars and syrups that are added to foods at the table or during processing or preparation (such as high fructose corn syrup in sweet- ened beverages and baked products). Although the body's response to sugars does not depend on whether they are naturally present in a food or added to the food, added sugars supply calories but few or no nutrients.

Consequently, it is important to choose carbohydrates wisely. Foods in the basic food groups that provide carbohydrates— vegetables, grains, and milk important sources of many nutrients. Choosing plenty of these foods, within the context of a calorie-controlled diet, can promote health and reduce chronic disease risk. However, the greater the consumption of foods containing large amounts of added sugars, the more difficult it is to consume enough nutrients without gaining weight. Consumption of added sugars provides calories while providing little, if any, of the essential nutrients.

DISCUSSION

The recommended dietary fiber intake is 14 grams per 1,000 calories consumed. Initially, some Americans will find it challenging to achieve this level of intake. However, making fiber-rich food choices more often will move people toward this goal and is likely to confer significant health benefits.

The majority of servings from the fruit group should come from whole fruit (fresh, frozen, canned, dried) rather than juice. Increasing the proportion of fruit that is eaten in the form of whole fruit rather than juice is desirable to increase fiber intake. However, inclusion of some juice, such as orange juice, can help meet recommended levels of potas- sium intake. Appendixes B-1 and B-8 list some of the best sources of potassium and dietary fiber, respectively.

Legumes— rich in fiber and should be consumed several times per week. They are considered part of both the vegetable group and the meat and beans group as they contain nutrients found in each of these food groups.

Consuming at least half the recommended grain servings as whole grains is important, for all ages, at each calorie level, to meet the fiber recommendation. Consuming at least 3 ounce-equivalents of whole grains per day can reduce the risk of coronary heart disease, may help with weight maintenance, and may lower risk for other chronic diseases. Thus, at lower calorie levels, adults should consume more than half (specifically, at least 3 ounce- equivalents) of whole grains per day, by substituting whole grains for refined grains. (See table 7 for a list of whole grains available in the United States.)

Diets rich in dietary fiber have been shown to have a number of beneficial effects.

KEY RECOMMENDATIONS

- Choose fiber-rich fruits, vegetables, and whole grains often.
- Choose and prepare foods and beverages with little added sugars or caloric sweeteners, such as amounts suggested by the USDA Food Guide and the DASH Eating Plan.
- Reduce the incidence of dental caries by practicing good oral hygiene and consuming sugar- and starch-containing foods and beverages less frequently.

Individuals who consume food or beverages high in added sugars tend to consume more calories than those who consume food or beverages low in added sugars; they also tend to consume lower amounts of micronutrients. Although more research is needed, available prospective studies show a positive association between the consumption of calorically sweetened beverages and weight gain. For this such as dry beans and peas reason, decreased intake of such foods, especially beverages with caloric sweeteners, is recommended to reduce calorie intake and help achieve recommended nutrient intakes and weight control.

Total discretionary calories should not exceed the allowance for any given calorie level, as shown in the USDA Food Guide (see ch. 2). The discretionary calorie allowance covers all calories from added sugars, alcohol, and the additional fat found in even moderate fat choices from the milk and meat group. For example, the 2,000- calorie pattern includes only about 267 discretionary calories. At 29 percent of calories from total fat (including 18 g of solid fat), if no alcohol is consumed, then only 8 teaspoons (32 g) of added sugars can be afforded. This is less than the amount in a typical 12-ounce calorically sweetened soft drink. If fat is decreased to 22 percent of calories, then 18 teaspoons (72 g) of added sugars is allowed. If fat is increased to 35 percent of calories, then no allowance remains for added sugars, even if alcohol is not consumed.

In some cases, small amounts of sugars added to nutrient- dense foods, such as breakfast cereals and reduced-fat milk products, may increase a person's intake of such foods by enhancing the palatability of these products, thus improving nutrient intake without contributing excessive calories. The major sources of added sugars are listed in table 13 (app. A-3 provides examples of how added sugars can fit into the discretionary calorie allowance).

...the greater the consumption of foods containing large amounts of added sugars, the more difficult it is to consume enough nutrients without gaining weight.

The Nutrition Facts Panel on the food label provides the amount of total sugars but does not list added sugars separately. People should examine the ingredient list to find out whether a food contains added sugars. The ingredient list is usually located under the Nutrition Facts Panel or on the side of a food label. Ingredients are listed in order of predominance, by weight; that is, the ingredient with the greatest contribution to the product weight is listed first and the ingredient contributing the least amount is listed last. Table 14 lists ingredients that are included in the term "added sugars". [1]

Sugars and starches contribute to dental caries by providing substrate for bacterial fermentation in the mouth. Thus, the frequency and duration of consumption of starches and sugars can be important factors because they increase exposure to cariogenic substrates. Drinking fluoridated water and/or using fluoride-containing dental hygiene products help reduce the risk of dental caries. Most bottled water is not fluoridated. With the increase in consumption of bottled water, there is concern that Americans may not be getting enough fluoride for maintenance of oral health. A combined approach of reducing the frequency and duration of exposure to fermentable carbohydrate intake and optimizing oral hygiene practices, such as drinking fluoridated water and brushing and flossing teeth, is the most effective way to reduce incidence of dental caries.

Considerations for Specific Population Groups

Older Adults

Dietary fiber is important for laxation. Since constipation may affect up to 20 percent of people over 65 years of age, older adults should choose to consume foods rich in dietary fiber. Other causes of constipation among this age group may include drug interactions with laxation and lack of appropriate hydration (see ch. 2).

Children

Carbohydrate intakes of children need special considerations with regard to obtaining sufficient amounts of fiber, avoiding excessive amounts of calories from added sugars, and preventing dental caries. Several cross-sectional surveys on U.S. children and adolescents have found inadequate dietary fiber intakes, which could be improved by increasing consumption of whole fruits, vegetables, and whole-grain products. Sugars can improve the palatability of foods and beverages that otherwise might not be consumed. This may explain why the consumption of sweetened dairy foods and beverages and presweetened cereals is positively associated with childrens' beverages with caloric sweeteners, sugars and sweets, and other sweetened foods that provide little or no nutrients are negatively associated with diet quality and can contribute to excessive energy intakes, sugars. affirming the importance of reducing added sugar intake substantially from current levels. Most of the studies of preschool children suggest a positive association between sucrose consumption and dental caries, though other factors (particularly infrequent brushing or not using fluoridated toothpaste) are more predictive of caries outcome than is sugar consumption.

Table 13. Major Sources of Added Sugars (Caloric Sweeteners) in the American Diet

Food groups that contribute more than 5 percent of the added sugars to the American diet in decreasing order.

Food Categories	Contribution to Added Sugars Intake (percent of total added sugars consumed)
Regular soft drinks	33.0
Sugars and candy	16.1
Cakes, cookies, pies	12.9
Fruit drinks (fruitades and fruit punch)	9.7
Dairy desserts and milk products (ice cream, sweetened yogurt, and sweetened milk)	8.6
Other grains (cinnamon toast and honey-nut waffles)	5.8

Source: Guthrie and Morton, Journal of the American Dietetic Association , 2000.

Table 14. Names for Added Sugars That Appear on Food Labels

Some of the names for added sugars that may be in processed foods and listed on the label ingredients list.

Brown sugar	Invert sugar
Corn sweetener	Lactose
Corn syrup	Maltose
Dextrose	Malt syrup
Fructose	Molasses
Fruit juice concentrates	Raw sugar
Glucose	Sucrose
High-fructose corn syrup	Sugar
Honey	Syrup

REFERENCES

[1] For information on amounts of added sugars in some common foods, see Krebs-Smith, SM. Choose beverages and foods to moderate your intake of sugars: measurement requires quantification. *The Journal of Nutrition (J Nutr)* **131**(2S-I): 527S-535S, 2001.

In: Dietary Guide   ISBN: 1-59454-654-1
Editor: Albert O. Gomber, pp. 77-82   © 2007 Nova Science Publishers, Inc.

Chapter 8

SODIUM AND POTASSIUM

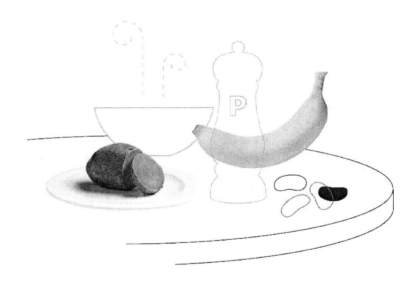

OVERVIEW

On average, the higher an individual's salt (sodium chloride) intake, the higher an individual's blood pressure. Nearly all Americans consume substantially more salt than they need. Decreasing salt intake is advisable to reduce the risk of elevated blood pressure. Keeping blood pressure in the normal range reduces an individual's risk of coronary heart disease, stroke, congestive heart failure, and kidney disease. Many American adults will develop hypertension (high blood pressure) during their lifetime. Lifestyle changes can prevent or delay the onset of high blood pressure and can lower elevated blood pressure. These changes include reducing salt intake, increasing potassium intake, losing excess body weight, increasing physical activity, and eating an overall healthful diet.

DISCUSSION

Salt is sodium chloride. Food labels list sodium rather than salt content. When reading a Nutrition Facts Panel on a food product, look for the sodium content. Foods that are low in sodium (less than 140 mg or 5 percent of the Daily Value [DV]) are low in salt.

Common sources of sodium found in the food supply are provided in figure 4. On average, the natural salt content of food accounts for only about 10 percent of total intake, while discretionary salt use (i.e., salt added at the table or while cooking) provides another 5 to 10 percent of total intake. Approximately 75 percent is derived from salt added by manufacturers. In addition, foods served by food establishments may be high in sodium. It is important to read the food label and determine the sodium content of food, which can vary by several hundreds of milligrams in similar foods. For example, the sodium content in regular tomato soup may be 700 mg per cup in one brand and 1,100 mg per cup in another brand. Reading labels, comparing sodium contents of foods, and purchasing the lower sodium brand may be one strategy to lower total sodium intake (see table 15 for examples of these foods).

An individual's preference for salt is not fixed. After consuming foods lower in salt for a period of time, taste for salt tends to decrease. Use of other flavorings may satisfy an individual's taste. While salt substitutes containing potassium chloride may be useful for some individuals, they can be harmful to people with certain medical conditions. These individuals should consult a healthcare provider before trying salt substitutes.

Discretionary salt use is fairly stable, even when foods offered are lower in sodium than typical foods consumed. When consumers are offered a lower sodium product, they typically do not add table salt to compensate for the lower sodium content, even when available. Therefore, any program for reducing the salt consumption of a population should concentrate primarily on reducing the salt used during food processing and on changes in food selection (e.g., more fresh, less-processed items, less sodium-dense foods) and preparation.

Lifestyle changes can prevent or delay the onset of high blood pressure and can lower elevated blood pressure.

KEY RECOMMENDATIONS

- Consume less than 2,300 mg (approximately 1 tsp of salt) of sodium per day.
- Choose and prepare foods with little salt. At the same time, consume potassium-rich foods, such as fruits and vegetables.

Key Recommendations for Specific Population Groups

- *Individuals with hypertension, blacks, and middle-aged and older adults.* Aim to consume no more than 1,500 mg of sodium per day, and meet the potassium recommendation (4,700 mg/day) with food.

Reducing salt intake is one of several ways that people may lower their blood pressure. The relationship between salt intake and blood pressure is direct and progressive without an apparent threshold. On average, the higher a person's, the higher the blood pressure. Reducing blood pressure, ideally to the normal range, reduces the risk of stroke, heart disease, heart failure, and kidney disease.

Another dietary measure to lower blood pressure is to consume a diet rich in potassium. A potassium-rich diet also blunts the effects of salt on blood pressure, may reduce the risk of developing kidney stones, and possibly decrease bone loss with age. The recommended intake of potassium for adolescents and adults is 4,700 mg/day. Recommended intakes for potassium for children 1 to 3 years of age is 3,000 mg/day, 4 to 8 years of age is 3,800 mg/day, and 9 to 13 years of age is 4,500 mg/day. Potassium should come from food sources. Fruits and vegetables, which are rich in potassium with its bicarbonate precursors, favorably affect acid-base metabolism, which may reduce risk of kidney stones and bone loss. Potassium-rich fruits and vegetables include leafy green vegetables, fruit from vines, and root vegetables. Meat, milk, and cereal products also contain potassium, but may not have the same effect on acid-base metabolism. Dietary sources of potassium are listed in table 5 and appendix B-1.

Considerations for Specific Population Groups

Individuals With Hypertension, Blacks, and Middle-Aged and Older Adults. Some individuals tend to be more salt sensitive than others, including people with hypertension, blacks, and middle-aged and older adults. Because blacks commonly have a relatively low intake of potassium and a high prevalence of elevated blood pressure and salt sensi-tivity, this population subgroup may especially benefit from an increased dietary intake of potassium. Dietary potassium can lower blood pressure and blunt the effects of salt on blood pressure in some individuals. While salt substitutes containing potassium chloride may be useful for some individuals, they can be harmful to people with certain medical conditions. These individuals should consult a healthcare provider before using salt substitutes.

The relative amounts of dietary sodium in the American diet.

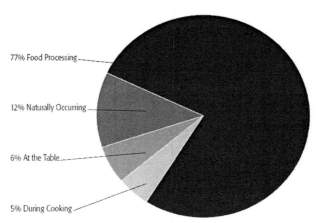

Source: Mattes RD, Donnelly D. Relative contributions of dietary sodium sources. *J Am Coll Nutr.* 1991 Aug;10(4):38393.

Figure 4. Sources of Dietary Sodium

Table 15. Range of Sodium Content for Selected F oods

The ranges of sodium content for selected foods available in the retail market.   This table is provided to e xemplify the importance of reading the food label to determine the sodium content of food, which can var y by several hundreds of milligrams in similar foods.

Food Group	Serving Size	Range (mg)
Breads, all types	1 oz	95-210
Frozen pizza, plain, cheese	4 oz	450-1200
Frozen vegetables, all types	$^1/_2$ c	2-160
Salad dressing, regular fat, all types	2 Tbsp	110-505
Salsa	2 Tbsp	150-240
Soup (tomato), reconstituted	8 oz	700-1260
Tomato juice	8 oz (~1 c)	340-1040
Potato chips[a]	1 oz (28.4 g)	120-180
Tortilla chips[a]	1 oz (28.4 g)	105-160
Pretzels[a]	1 oz (28.4 g)	290-560

[a] All snack foods are regular flavor, salted.

Source: Agricultural Research Service Nutrient Database for Standard Reference, Release 17 and recent manufacturers label data from retail market surveys. Serving sizes were standardized to be comparable among brands within a food. Pizza and bread slices vary in size and weight across brands.

Note: None of the e xamples provided were labeled low-sodium products.

In: Dietary Guide   ISBN: 1-59454-654-1
Editor: Albert O. Gomber, pp. 83-87   © 2007 Nova Science Publishers, Inc.

Chapter 9

ALCOHOLIC BEVERAGES

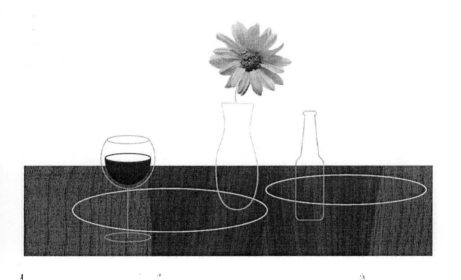

OVERVIEW

The consumption of alcohol can have beneficial or harmful effects depending on the amount consumed, age and other characteristics of the person consuming the alcohol, and specifics of the situation. In 2002, 55 percent of U.S. adults were current drinkers. Forty-five percent of U.S. adults do not drink any alcohol at all. [1] Abstention is an important option.

Fewer Americans consume alcohol today as compared to 50 to 100 years ago.

The hazards of heavy alcohol consumption are well known and include increased risk of liver cirrhosis, hyper- tension, cancers of the upper gastrointestinal tract, injury, violence, and death. Moreover, certain individuals who are more susceptible to the harmful effects of alcohol should not drink at all. In addition, alcohol should be avoided by those participating in activities that require attention, skill, and/or coordination.

Alcohol may have beneficial effects when consumed in moderation. The lowest all-cause mortality occurs at an intake of one to two drinks per day. The lowest coronary heart disease mortality also occurs at an intake of one to two drinks per day. Morbidity and mortality are highest among those drinking large amounts of alcohol.

DISCUSSION

Alcoholic beverages supply calories but few essential nutrients (see table 16). As a result, excessive alcohol consumption makes it difficult to ingest sufficient nutri- ents within an individual's daily calorie allotment and to maintain a healthy weight. Although the consumption of one to two alcoholic beverages per day is not associated with macronutrient or micronutrient deficiencies or with overall dietary quality, heavy drinkers may be at risk of malnutrition if the calories derived from alcohol are substi- tuted for those in nutritious foods.

The majority of American adults consume alcohol. Those who do so should drink alcoholic beverages in moderation. Moderation is defined as the consumption of up to one drink per day for women and up to two drinks per day for men. Twelve fluid ounces of regular beer, 5 fluid ounces of wine, or 1.5 fluid ounces of 80-proof distilled spirits count as one drink for purposes of explaining moderation. This definition of moderation is not intended as an average over several days but rather as the amount consumed on any single day.

The effect of alcohol consumption varies depending on the amount consumed and an and circumstances. Alcoholic beverages are harmful when consumed in excess. Excess alcohol consumption alters judgment and can lead to dependency or addiction and other serious health problems such as cirrhosis of the liver, inflammation of the pancreas, and damage to the heart and brain. Even less than heavy consumption of alcohol is associated with significant risks. Consuming more than one drink per day for women and two drinks per day for men increases the risk for motor vehicle accidents, other injuries, high blood pressure, stroke, violence, some types of cancer, and suicide. Compared with women who do not drink, women who consume one drink per day appear to have a slightly higher risk of breast cancer.

Alcoholic beverages supply calories but few essential nutrients.

KEY RECOMMENDATIONS

- Those who choose to drink alcoholic beverages should do so sensibly and in moderation – defined as the consumption of up to one drink per day for women and to up to two drinks per day for men.
- Alcoholic beverages should not be consumed by some individuals, including those who cannot restrict their alcohol intake, women of childbearing age who may become pregnant, pregnant and lactating women, children and adolescents, individuals taking medications that can interact with alcohol, and those with specific medical conditions.
- Alcoholic beverages should be avoided by individuals engaging in activities that require attention, skill, or coordination, such as driving or operating machinery.

Studies suggest adverse effects even at moderate alcohol consumption levels in specific situations and individuals. Individuals in some situations should avoid alcohol characteristics who plan to drive, operate machinery, or take part in other activities that require attention, skill, or coordination. Some people, including children and adolescents, women of childbearing age who may become pregnant, pregnant and lactating women, individuals who cannot restrict alcohol intake, individuals taking medications that can interact with alcohol, and individuals with specific medical conditions should not drink at all. Even moderate drinking during pregnancy may have behavioral or developmental consequences for the baby. Heavy drinking during pregnancy can produce a range of behavioral and psychosocial problems, malformation, and mental retardation in the baby.

Table 16. Calories in Selected Alcoholic Beverages

This table is a guide to estimate the caloric intake from various alcoholic beverages. An example serving volume and the calories in that drink are shown for beer, wine, and distilled spirits. Higher alcohol content (higher percent alcohol or higher proof) and mixing alcohol with other beverages, such as calorically sweetened soft drinks, tonic water, fruit juice, or cream, increases the amount of calories in the beverage. Alcoholic beverages supply calories but provide few essential nutrients.

Beverage	Approximate Calories Per 1 Fluid Oz[a]	Example Serving Volume	Approximate Total Calories[b]
Beer (regular)	12	12 oz	144
Beer (light)	9	12 oz	108
White wine	20	5 oz	100
Red wine	21	5 oz	105
Sweet dessert wine	47	3 oz	141
80 proof distilled spirits (gin, rum, vodka, whiskey)	64	1.5 oz	96

[a] Source: Agricultural Research Service (ARS) Nutrient Database for Standard Reference (SR), Release 17. (http://www.nal.usda.gov/fnic/foodcomp/index.html) Calories are calculated to the nearest whole number per 1 fluid oz.

b The total calories and alcohol content vary depending on the brand. Moreover, adding mixers to an alcoholic beverage can contribute calories in addition to the calories from the alcohol itself.

Moderate alcohol consumption may have beneficial health effects in some individuals. In middle-aged and older adults, a daily intake of one to two alcoholic beverages per day is associated with the lowest all-cause mortality. More specifically, compared to non-drinkers, adults who consume one to two alcoholic beverages a day appear to have a lower risk of coronary heart disease. In contrast, among younger adults alcohol consumption appears to provide little, if any, health benefit, and alcohol use among young adults is associated with a higher risk of traumatic injury and death. As noted previously, a number of strategies reduce the risk of chronic disease, including a healthful diet, physical activity, avoidance of smoking, and maintenance of a healthy weight. Furthermore, it is not recommended that anyone begin drinking or drink more frequently on the basis of health considerations.

REFERENCES

[1]   Behavioral Risk Factor Surveillance System, Surveillance for Certain Health Behaviors Among Selected Local Areas—United *MMWR*, **53**, No SS- States, 05. http://www.cdc.gov/brfss/.

In: Dietary Guide
Editor: Albert O. Gomber, pp. 89-93

ISBN: 1-59454-654-1
© 2007 Nova Science Publishers, Inc.

Chapter 10

FOOD SAFETY

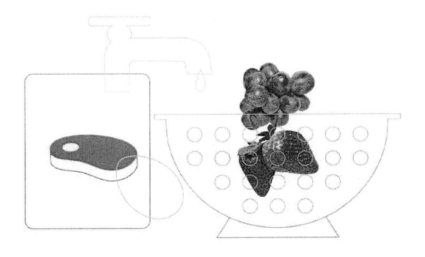

OVERVIEW

Avoiding foods that are contaminated with harmful bacteria, viruses, parasites, toxins, and chemical and physical contaminants are vital for healthful eating. The signs and symptoms of foodborne illness range from gastrointestinal symptoms, such as upset stomach, diarrhea, fever, vomiting, abdominal cramps, and dehydration, to more severe systemic illness, such as paralysis and meningitis. It is estimated that every year about 76 million people in the United States become ill from pathogens in food; of these, about 5,000 die. Consumers can take simple measures to reduce their risk of foodborne illness, especially in the home.

DISCUSSION

The most important food safety problem is microbial foodborne illness. All those who handle food, including farmers, food producers, individuals who work in markets and food service establishments, and other food preparers, have a responsibility to keep food as safe as possible. To keep food safe, people who prepare food should clean hands, food contact surfaces, and fruits and vegetables; separate raw, cooked, and ready-to-eat foods; cook foods to a safe internal temperature; chill perishable food promptly; and defrost food properly. For more important information on cooking, cleaning, separating, and chilling, see www.fightbac.org.

Consumers can take simple measures to reduce their risk of foodborne illness, especially in the home.

When preparing and consuming food, it is essential to wash hands often, particularly before and after preparing food, especially after handling raw meat, poultry, eggs, or seafood. A good hand washing protocol includes wetting hands; applying soap; rubbing hands vigorously together for 20 seconds; rinsing hands thoroughly under clean, running warm water; and drying hands completely using a clean disposable or cloth towel.

Washing may be the only method that consumers have to reduce pathogen load on fresh produce that will not be either peeled or subsequently cooked. A good protocol for washing fresh fruits and vegetables includes removing and discarding outer leaves, washing produce just before cooking or eating, washing under running potable water, scrubbing with a clean brush or with hands, and drying the fruits or vegetables using a clean disposable or cloth towel. Free moisture on produce may promote survival and growth of microbial populations. Therefore, drying the food is critical if the item will not be eaten or cooked right away.

People should read the labels of bagged produce to deter- mine if it is ready-to-eat. Ready-to-eat, prewashed bagged produce can be used without further washing if kept refrigerated and used by the "use-by" date. If desired, prewashed, ready-to-eat produce can be washed again. Raw meat and poultry should not be washed because this creates the danger of cross-contamination and is not necessary. Washing these foods can allow most bacteria that are present on the surface of the meat or poultry to spread to ready-to-eat foods, kitchen utensils, and counter surfaces.

KEY RECOMMENDATIONS

To avoid microbial foodborne illness:

- Clean hands, food contact surfaces, and fruits and vegetables. Meat and poultry should *not* be washed or rinsed.
- Separate raw, cooked, and ready-to-eat foods while shopping, preparing, or storing foods.
- Cook foods to a safe temperature to kill microorganisms.
- Chill (refrigerate) perishable food promptly and defrost foods properly.
- Avoid raw (unpasteurized) milk or any products made from unpasteurized milk, raw or partially cooked eggs or foods containing raw eggs, raw or undercooked meat and poultry, unpasteurized juices, and raw sprouts.

Key Recommendations for Specific Population Groups

- *Infants and young children, pregnant women, older adults, and those who are immunocompromised.* Do not eat or drink raw (unpasteurized) milk or any products made from unpasteurized milk, raw or partially cooked eggs or foods containing raw eggs, raw or undercooked meat and poultry, raw or undercooked fish or shellfish, unpasteurized juices, and raw sprouts.
- *Pregnant women, older adults, and those who are immunocompromised:* Only eat certain deli meats and frankfurters that have been reheated to steaming hot.

It is important to separate raw, cooked, and ready-to-eat foods while shopping, preparing, or storing. This prevents cross-contamination from one food to another. In addition, refrigerator surfaces can become contaminated from high- risk foods such as raw meats, poultry, fish, uncooked hot dogs, certain deli meats, or raw vegetables. If not cleaned, contaminated refrigerator surfaces can, in turn, serve as a vehicle for contaminating other foods. -

Uncooked and undercooked meat, poultry and eggs and egg products are potentially unsafe. Raw meat, poultry and eggs should always be cooked to a safe internal temperature (see fig. 5). The best way to tell if meat, poultry and egg dishes are cooked safely is to use a food thermometer. Leftover refrigerator foods should also be reheated to the proper internal temperature. Bacteria grow most rapidly in the range of 40 F and 140 F. To keep food out of this danger zone, keep cold food cold (below 40 F) and hot food hot (above 140 F). Figure 5 provides information for temperature rules for proper cooking and food handling. Proper cooking makes most uncooked foods safe.

The refrigerator should be set at no higher than 40 F and the freezer at 0 F, and these temperatures should be checked with an appliance thermometer. Refrigerated leftovers may become unsafe within 3 to 4 days. Despite the appearance of a food, it may not be safe to eat. Not all bacterial growth causes a food's surface to discolor or smell bad. It may be unsafe to taste fresh or leftover food items when there is any doubt about their safety. Safe disposal of the food is indicated if there is a question about whether or not a food is safe to eat. If in doubt - throw it out."

Considerations for Specific Population Groups Some people may be at high risk for developing foodborne illness. These include pregnant women and their fetuses, young children, older adults, people with weakened immune systems, and individuals with certain chronic illnesses. These people should pay extra attention to food safety advice.

For example, pregnant women, and older adults, and those 40°F) who are immunocompromised are at risk of developing listeriosis, a potentially life-threatening illness caused by the bacterium *Listeria monocytogenes*. Some deli meats and frankfurters that have not been reheated to steaming hot and some ready-to-eat foods are associated with liste- 40°F riosis and pose a high-risk to certain individuals. All these foods should be heated to a safe internal temperature. In addition, these individuals should take special care not to eat or drink raw (unpasteurized) milk or any products made from unpasteurized milk (such as some soft cheeses), raw or partially cooked eggs or foods containing raw eggs, surface to discolor or raw or undercooked meat and poultry, unpasteurized juices, and raw sprouts. They should also avoid raw or undercooked fish or shellfish.

New information on food safety is constantly emerging. Recommendations and precautions for people at high risk are updated as scientists learn more about preventing foodborne illness. Individuals in high-risk categories should seek guidance from a healthcare provider. In addition, up- to-date information is available at the Government's food safety website at www.foodsafety.gov.

Safe cooking and holding temperature for foods. Bacteria multiply rapidly between 40°F and 140°F, doubling in number in as a little as 20 minutes. To keep food out of this danger zone, keep cold food cold and hot food hot. Keep food cold in the refrigerator, in coolers or on the service line on ice. Set your refrigerator no higher than 40°F and the freezer at 0°F. Keep hot food in the oven, in heated chafing dishes, or in preheated steam tables, warming trays, and/or slow cookers. Use a clean thermometer that measures the internal temperature of cooked food, to make sure that meat, poultry and casseroles are cooked to the temperatures as indicated in the figure.

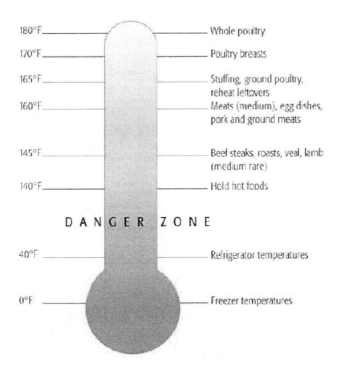

Figure 5. Temperature Rules for Safe Cooking and Handling of Foods

In: Dietary Guide
Editor: Albert O. Gomber, pp. 95-121

ISBN: 1-59454-654-1
© 2007 Nova Science Publishers, Inc.

APPENDICES

APPENDIX A. EATING PATTERNS

Appendix A-1: The DASH Eating Plan at 1,600-, 2,000-, 2600-, and 3,100-Calorie Levels [a]

The DASH eating plan is based on 1,600, 2,000, 2,600 and 3,100 calories. The number of daily servings in a food group vary depending on caloric needs (see Table 3 on page 12 to determine caloric needs). This chart can aid in planning menus and food selection in restaurants and grocery stores.

Food Groups	1,600 Calories	2,000 Calories	2,600 Calories	3,100 Calories	Serving Sizes	Examples and Notes	Significance of Each Food Group to the DASH Eating Plan
Grains[b]	6 servings	7-8 servings	10-11 servings	12—13 servings	1 slice bread, 1 oz dry cereal, 1/2 cup cooked rice, pasta, or cereal[c]	Whole wheat bread, English muffin, pita bread, bagel, cereals, grits, oatmeal, crackers, unsalted pretzels, and popcorn	Major sources of energy and fiber
Vegetables	3-4 serving	4-5 servings	5—6 servings	6 servings	1 cup raw leafy vegetable 1/2 cup cooked vegetable 6 oz vegetable juice	Tomatoes, potatoes carrots, green peas, squash, broccoli, turnip greens, collards, kale, spinach, artichokes, green beans, lima beans, sweetpotatoes	Rich sources of potassium, magnesium, and fiber
Fruits	4 servings	4-5 servings	5—6 servings	6 servings	6 oz fruit juice 1 medium fruit 1/4 cup dried fruit 1/2 cup fresh, frozen, or canned fruit	dates, grapes, oranges, orange juice, grapefruit, grapefruit juice, mangoes, melons, peaches, pineapples, prunes, raisins, strawberries, tangerines	Important sources of potassium, magnesium, and fiber
Low-fat or fat-free dairy foods	2-3 servings	2—3 servings	3 servings	3—4 servings	8 oz milk 1 cup yogurt 1 1/2 oz cheese	Fat-free or low-fat milk, fat-free or low-fat buttermilk, fat-free or low-fat regular or frozen yogurt, low-fat and fat-free cheese	Major sources of calcium and protein
Meat, poultry, fish	1-2 servings	2 or less servings	2 servings	2-3 servings	3 oz cooked meats, poultry, or fish	Select only lean; trim away visible fats; broil, roast, or boil instead of frying; remove skin from poultry	Rich sources of protein and magnesium

Nuts, seeds, legumes	3-4 servings/ week		1 serving	$1/3$ cup or $1 1/2$ oz nuts 2 Tbsp or $1/2$ oz seeds $1/2$ cup cooked dry beans or peas	Almonds, filberts, mixed nuts, peanuts, walnuts, sunflower seeds, kidney beans, lentils	Rich sources of energy, magnesium, potassium, protein, and fiber
Fat and oils[d]	2 servings	2-3 servings	4 servings	1 tsp soft margarine 1 Tbsp low-fat mayonnaise 2 Tbsp light salad dressing 1 tsp vegetable oil	Soft margarine, low-fat mayonnaise, light salad dressing, vegetable oil (such as olive, corn, canola, or safflower)	DASH has 27 percent of calories as fat (low in saturated fat), including fat in or added to foods
Sweets	0 servings	5 servings/ week	2 servings	1 Tbsp sugar 1 Tbsp jelly or jam $1/2$ oz jelly beans 8 oz lemonade	Maple syrup, sugar, jelly, jam, fruit-flavored gelatin, jelly beans, hard candy, fruit punch sorbet, ices	Sweets should be low in fat

[a] NIH publication No. 03-4082; Karanja NM et al. *JADA* 8:S19—27, 1999.
[b] Whole grains are recommended for most servings to meet fiber recommendations.
[c] Equals $1/2$- $1/4$ cups, depending on cereal type. Check the product's Nutrition Facts Label.
[d] Serving; 1 Tbsp of a fat-free dressing

Fat content changes serving counts for fats and oils: For example, 1 Tbsp of regular salad dressing equals 1 serving; 1 Tbsp of a low-fat dressing equals $1/2$ serving; 1 Tbsp of a fat-free dressing equals 0 servings.

Appendix A2. USDA Food Guide

The suggested amounts of food to consume from the basic food groups, subgroups, and oils to meet recommended nutrient intakes at 1 2 different calorie levels. Nutrient and energy contributions from each group are calculated according to the nutrientdense forms of foods in each group (e.g., lean meats and fatfree milk). The table also sho ws the discretionary calorie allowance that can be accommodated within each calorie le vel, in addition to the suggested amounts of nutrientdense forms of foods in each group.

Daily Amount of Food From Each Group (vegetable subgroup amounts are per week)

Calorie Level	1,000	1,200	1,400	1,600	1,800	2,000	2,200	2,400	2,600	2,800	3,000	3,200
Food Group[1]	Food group amounts shown in cup (c) or ounce-equivalents (oz-eq), with number of servings (srv) in parentheses when it differs from the other units. See note for quantity equivalents for foods in each group.[2] Oils are shown in grams (g).											
Fruits	1 c (2 srv)	1 c (2 srv)	1.5 c (3 srv)	1.5 c (3 srv)	1.5 c (3 srv)	2 c (4 srv)	2 c (4 srv)	2 c (4 srv)	2 c (4 srv)	2.5 c (5 srv)	2.5 c (5 srv)	2.5 c (5 srv)
Vegetables[3]	1 c (2 srv)	1.5 c (3 srv)	1.5 c (3 srv)	2 c (4 srv)	2.5 c (5 srv)	2.5 c (5 srv)	3 c (6 srv)	3 c (6 srv)	3.5 c (7 srv)	3.5 c (7 srv)	4 c (8 srv)	4 c (8 srv)
Dark green veg.	1 c/wk	1.5 c/wk	1.5 c/wk	2 c/wk	3 c/wk	3 c/wk	3 c/wk	3 c/wk	3 c/wk	3 c/wk	3 c/wk	3 c/wk
Orange veg.	.5 c/wk	1 c/wk	1 c/wk	1.5 c/wk	2 c/wk	2 c/wk	2 c/wk	2 c/wk	2.5 c/wk	2.5 c/wk	2.5 c/wk	2.5 c/wk
Legumes	.5 c/wk	1 c/wk	1 c/wk	2.5 c/wk	3 c/wk	3 c/wk	3 c/wk	3 c/wk	3.5 c/wk	3.5 c/wk	3.5 c/wk	3.5 c/wk
Starchy veg.	1.5 c/wk	2.5 c/wk	2.5 c/wk	2.5 c/wk	3 c/wk	3 c/wk	6 c/wk	6 c/wk	7 c/wk	7 c/wk	9 c/wk	9 c/wk
Other veg.	3.5 c/wk	4.5 c/wk	4.5 c/wk	5.5 c/wk	6.5 c/wk	6.5 c/wk	7 c/wk	7 c/wk	8.5 c/wk	8.5 c/wk	10 c/wk	10 c/wk
Grains[4]	3 oz-eq	4 oz-eq	5 oz-eq	5 oz-eq	6 oz-eq	6 oz-eq	7 oz-eq	8 oz-eq	9 oz-eq	10 oz-eq	10 oz-eq	10 oz-eq
Whole grains	1.5	2	2.5	3	3	3	3.5	4	4.5	5	5	5
Other grains	1.5	2	2.5	2	3	3	3.5	4	4.5	5	5	5
Lean meat and beans	2 oz-eq	3 oz-eq	4 oz-eq	5 oz-eq	5 oz-eq	5.5 oz-eq	6 oz-eq	6.5 oz-eq	6.5 oz-eq	7 oz-eq	7 oz-eq	7 oz-eq
Milk	2 c	2 c	2 c	3 c	3 c	3 c	3 c	3 c	3 c	3 c	3 c	3 c
Oils[5]	15 g	17 g	17 g	22 g	24 g	27 g	29 g	31 g	34 g	36 g	44 g	51 g
Discretionary calorie allowance[6]	165	171	171	132	195	267	290	362	410	426	512	648

Notes for Appendix A-2:

[1] Food items included in each group and subgroup:

Fruits	All fresh, frozen, canned, and dried fruits and fruit juices: for example, oranges and orange juice, apples and apple juice, bananas, grapes, melons, berries, raisins. In developing the food patterns, only fruits and juices with no added sugars or fats were used. *See note 6 on discretionary calories if products with added sugars or fats are consumed.*
Vegetables	In developing the food patterns, only vegetables with no added fats or sugars were used. *See note 6 on discretionary calories if products with added fats or sugars are consumed.*
• Dark green vegetables	All fresh, frozen, and canned dark green vegetables, cooked or raw: for example, broccoli; spinach; romaine; collard, turnip,and mustard greens.
• Orange vegetables	All fresh, frozen, and canned orange and deep yellow vegetables, cooked or raw: for example, carrots, sweetpotatoes, winter squash, and pumpkin.
• Legumes	All cooked dry beans and peas and soybean products: for example, pinto beans, kidney beans, lentils, chickpeas, tofu.
(dry beans and peas)	(See comment under meat and beans group about counting legumes in the vegetable or the meat and beans group.)
• Starchy vegetables	All fresh, frozen, and canned starchy vegetables: for example, white potatoes, corn, green peas.
• Other vegetables	All fresh, frozen, and canned other vegetables, cooked or raw: for example, tomatoes, tomato juice, lettuce, green beans, onions.
Grains	In developing the food patterns, only grains in low-fat and low-sugar forms were used. *See note 6 on discretionary calories if products that are higher in fat and/or added sugars are consumed.*
• Whole grains	All whole-grain products and whole grains used as ingredients: for example, whole-wheat and rye breads, whole-grain cereals and crackers, oatmeal, and brown rice.
• Other grains	All refined grain products and refined grains used as ingredients: for example, white breads, enriched grain cereals and crackers, enriched pasta, white rice.
Meat, poultry, fish, dry beans, eggs, and nuts (meat & beans)	All meat, poultry, fish, dry beans and peas, eggs, nuts, seeds. Most choices should be lean or low-fat. *See note 6 on discretionary calories if higher fat products are consumed* Dry beans and peas and soybean products are considered part of this group as well as the vegetable group, but should be counted in one group only.
Milk, yogurt, and cheese (milk)	All milks, yogurts, frozen yogurts, dairy desserts, cheeses (except cream cheese), including lactose-free and lactose-reduced products. Most choices should be fat-free or low-fat. In developing the food patterns, only fat-free milk was used. *See note 6 on discretionary calories if low-fat, reduced-fat, or whole milk or milk products products that contain added sugars are consumed.* Calcium-for tified soy beverages are an option for those who want a non-dairy calcium source.

2 Quantity equivalents for each food group:

Grains	The following each count as 1 ounce-equivalent (1 serving) of grains: $\frac{1}{2}$ cup cooked rice, pasta, or cooked cereal; 1 ounce dr y pasta or rice; 1 slice bread; 1 small muffin (1 oz); 1 cup ready-to-eat cereal flakes.
Fruits and vegetables	The following each count as 1 cup (2 servings) of fruits or vegetables: 1 cup cut-up raw or cooked fruit or vegetable, 1 cup fruit or vegetable juice, 2 cups leafy salad greens.
Meat and beans	The following each count as 1 ounce-equivalent: 1 ounce lean meat, poultry, or fish; 1 egg; $\frac{1}{4}$ cup cooked dry beans or tofu; 1 Tbsp peanut butter; $\frac{1}{2}$ ounce nuts or seeds.
Milk	The following each count as 1 cup (1 serving) of milk: 1 cup milk or yogurt, 1 $\frac{1}{2}$ ounces natural cheese such as Cheddar cheese or 2 ounces processed cheese. Discretionary calories must be counted for all choices, except fat-free milk.

3 Explanation of vegetable subgroup amounts: Vegetable subgroup amounts are shown in this table as weekly amounts, because it would be difficult for consumers to select foods from each subgroup daily. A daily amount that is one-seventh of the weekly amount listed is used in calculations of nutrient and energy levels in each pattern.

4 Explanation of grain subgroup amounts: The whole grain subgroup amounts shown in this table represent at least three 1-ounce servings and one-half of the total amount as whole grains for all calorie levels of 1,600 and above. This is the minimum suggested amount of whole grains to consume as part of the food patterns. More whole grains up to all of the grains recommended may be selected, with offsetting decreases in the amounts of other (enriched) grains. In patterns designed for younger children (1,000, 1,200, and 1 ,400 calories), one-half of the total amount of grains is shown as whole grains.

5 Explanation of oils: Oils (including soft margarine with zero *trans* fat) shown in this table represent the amounts that are added to foods during processing, cooking, or at the table. Oils and soft margarines include vegetable oils and soft vegetable oil table spreads that have no *trans* fats. The amounts of oils listed in this table are not considered to be par t of discretionary calories because they are a major source of the vitamin E and polyunsaturated fatty acids, including the essential fatty acids, in the food pattern. In contrast, solid fats are listed separately in the discretionary calorie table (appendix A-3) because, compared with oils, they are higher in saturated fatty acids and lower in vitamin E and polyunsaturated and monounsaturated fatty acids, including essential fatty acids. The amounts of each type of fat in the food intake pattern were based on 60% oils and/or soft margarines with no *trans* fats and 40% solid fat. The amounts in typical American diets are about 42% oils or soft margarines and about 58% solid fats.

6 Explanation of discretionary calorie allowance: The discretionary calorie allowance is the remaining amount of calories in each food pattern after selecting the specified number of nutrient-dense forms of foods in each food group. The number of discretionar y calories

assumes that food items in each food group are selected in nutrient-dense forms (that is, forms that are fat-free or lo w-fat and that contain no added sugars). Solid fat and sugar calories always need to be counted as discretionary calories, as in the following examples:
• The fat in low-fat, reduced fat, or whole milk or milk products or cheese and the sugar and fat in chocolate milk, ice cream, pudding, etc.
• The fat in higher fat meats (e.g., ground beef with more than 5% fat by weight, poultry with skin, higher fat luncheon meats, sausages)
• The sugars added to fruits and fruit juices with added sugars or fruits canned in syrup
• The added fat and/or sugars in vegetables prepared with added fat or sugars
• The added fats and/or sugars in grain products containing higher levels of fats and/or sugars (e.g., sweetened cereals, higher fat crackers, pies and other pastries, cakes, cookies)

Total discretionary calories should be limited to the amounts shown in the table at each calorie level. The number of discretionary calories is lower in the 1,600-calorie pattern than in the 1,000-, 1,200-, and 1,400-calorie patterns. These lower calorie patterns are designed to meet the nutrient needs of children 2 to 8 years old. The nutrient goals for the 1,600-calorie pattern are set to meet the needs of adult women, which are higher and require that more calories be used in selections from the basic food groups. Additional information about discretionar y calories, including an example of the division of these calories between solid fats and added sugars, is provided in appendix A-3.

Appendix A-3. Discretionary Calorie Allowance in the USDA Food Guide

The discretionary calorie allowance is the remaining amount of calories in each calorie level after nutrient-dense forms of foods in each food group are selected. This table shows the number of discretionary calories remaining in each calorie level if nutrient-dense foods are selected. Those trying to lose weight may choose not to use discretionary calories. For those wanting to maintain their weight, discretionary calories may be used to increase the amount of food selected from each food group; to consume foods that are not in the lowest fat form (such as 2% milk or medium-fat meat) or that contain added sugars; to add oil, fat, or sugars to foods; or to consume alcohol. The table shows an example of how these calories may be divided between solid fats and added sugars.

Discretionary calories that remain at each calorie level

Food Guide calorie level	1,000	1,200	1,400	1,600	1,800	2,000	2,200	2,400	2,600	2,800	3,000	3,200
Discretionary calories[1]	165	171	171	132	195	267	290	362	410	426	512	648

Example of division of discretionary calories: Solid fats are shown in grams (g); added sugars in grams (g) and teaspoons (tsp).

Solid fats[2]	11 g	14 g	14 g	11 g	15 g	18 g	19 g	22 g	24 g	24 g	29 g	34 g
Added sugars[3]	20 g (5 tsp)	16 g (4 tsp)	16 g (4 tsp)	12 g (3 tsp)	20 g (5 tsp)	32 g (8 tsp)	36 g (9 tsp)	48 g (12 tsp)	56 g (14 tsp)	60 g (15 tsp)	72g (18 tsp)	96 g (24 tsp)

1   Discretionary calories: In developing the Food Guide, food items in nutrient-dense forms (that is, forms that are fat-free or low-fat and that contain no added sugars) were used. The number of discretionary calories assumes that food items in each food group are selected in nutrient-dense forms. Solid fat and sugar calories always need to be counted as discretionar y calories, as in the following examples:

    The fat in low-fat, reduced fat, or whole milk or milk products or cheese and the sugar and fat in chocolate milk, ice cream, pudding, etc.

    The fat in higher fat meats (e.g., ground beef with more than 5% fat by weight, poultr y with skin, higher fat luncheon meats, sausages)

    The sugars added to fruits and fruit juices with added sugars or fruits canned in syrup

    The added fat and/or sugars in vegetables prepared with added fat or sugars

    The added fats and/or sugars in grain products containing higher levels of fats and/or sugars (e.g., sweetened cereals, higher fat crackers, pies and other pastries, cakes, cookies)

    Total discretionary calories should be limited to the amounts shown in the table at each calorie level. The number of discretionary calories is lower in the 1,600 calorie pattern than in the 1,000, 1,200, and 1,400-calorie patterns. These lower calorie patterns are designed to meet the nutrient needs of children 2 to 8 years old. The nutrient goals for the 1,600 calorie pattern are set to meet the needs of adult women, which are higher and require that more calories be used in selections from the basic food groups. The calories assigned to discretionar y calories may be used to increase intake from the basic food groups; to select foods from these groups that are higher in fat or with added sugars; to add oils, solid fats, or sugars to foods or beverages; or to consume alcohol. See note 2 on limits for solid fats.

2   Solid fats: Amounts of solid fats listed in the table represent about 7 to 8% of calories from saturated fat. Foods in each food group are represented in their lowest fat forms, such as fat-free milk and skinless chicken. Solid fats shown in this table represent the amounts of fats that may be added in cooking or at the table, and fats consumed when higher fat items are selected from the food groups (e.g., whole milk instead of fat-free milk, chicken with skin, or cookies instead of bread), without exceeding the recommended limits on saturated fat intake. Solid fats include meat and poultry fats eaten either as part of the meat or poultry product or separately; milk fat such as that in whole milk, cheese, and butter; shortenings used in baked products; and hard margarines.

    Solid fats and oils are separated because their fatty acid compositions differ. Solid fats are higher in saturated fatty acids, and commonly consumed oils and soft margarines with no *trans* fats are higher in vitamin E and polyunsaturated and monounsaturated fatty acids, including essential fatty acids. Oils listed in appendix A-2 are not considered to be par t of the discretionary calorie allowance because they are a major source of the essential fatty acids and vitamin E in the food pattern.

    The gram weights for solid fats are the amounts of these products that can be included in the pattern and are not identical to the amount of lipids in these items, because some products (margarines, butter) contain water or other ingredients, in addition to lipids.

3   Added sugars: Added sugars are the sugars and syrups added to foods and beverages in processing or preparation, not the naturally occurring sugars in fruits or milk. The amounts of added sugars suggested in the example are NOT specific recommendations for amounts

of added sugars to consume, but rather represent the amounts that can be included at each calorie level without over- consuming calories. The suggested amounts of added sugars may be helpful as part of the Food Guide to allow for some sweetened foods or beverages, without exceeding energy needs. This use of added sugars as a calorie balance requires two assumptions: (1) that selections are made from all food groups in accordance with the suggested amounts and (2) that additional fats are used in the amounts shown, which, together with the fats in the core food groups, represent about 27-30% of calories from fat.

APPENDIX B. FOOD SOURCES OF SELECTED NUTRIENTS

Appendix B1. Food Sources of Potassium

Food Sources of Potassium ranked by milligrams of potassium per standard amount, also sho wing calories in the standard amount. (The AI for adults is 4,700 mg/day potassium.)

Food, Standard Amount	Potassium (mg)	Calories
Sweetpotato, baked, 1 potato (146 g)	694	131
Tomato paste, ¼ cup	664	54
Beet greens, cooked, ½ cup	655	19
Potato, baked, flesh, 1 potato (156 g)	610	145
White beans, canned, ½ cup	595	153
Yogurt, plain, non-fat, 8-oz container	579	127
Tomato puree, ½ cup	549	48
Clams, canned, 3 oz	534	126
Yogurt, plain, low-fat, 8-oz container	531	143
Prune juice, ¾ cup	530	136
Carrot juice, ¾ cup	517	71
Blackstrap molasses, 1 Tbsp	498	47
Halibut, cooked, 3 oz	490	119
Soybeans, green, cooked, ½ cup	485	127
Tuna, yellowfin, cooked, 3 oz	484	118
Lima beans, cooked, ½ cup	484	104
Winter squash, cooked, ½ cup	448	40
Soybeans, mature, cooked, ½ cup	443	149
Rockfish, Pacific, cooked, 3 oz	442	103
Cod, Pacific, cooked, 3 oz	439	89
Bananas, 1 medium	422	105
Spinach, cooked, ½ cup	419	21
Tomato juice, ¾ cup	417	31
Tomato sauce, ½ cup	405	39
Peaches, dried, uncooked, ¼ cup	398	96
Prunes, stewed, ½ cup	398	133
Milk, non-fat, 1 cup	382	83
Pork chop, center loin, cooked, 3 oz	382	197
Apricots, dried, uncooked, ¼ cup	378	78
Rainbow trout, farmed, cooked, 3 oz	375	144
Pork loin, center rib (roasts), lean, roasted, 3 oz	371	190
Buttermilk, cultured, low-fat, 1 cup	370	98
Cantaloupe, ¼ medium	368	47
1%–2% milk, 1 cup	366	102–122
Honeydew melon, ⅛ medium	365	58
Lentils, cooked, ½ cup	365	115
Plantains, cooked, ½ cup slices	358	90
Kidney beans, cooked, ½ cup	358	112
Orange juice, ¾ cup	355	85
Split peas, cooked, ½ cup	355	116
Yogurt, plain, whole milk, 8 oz container	352	138

Source: Nutrient values from Agricultural Research Ser vice (ARS) Nutrient Database for Standard Reference, Release 17. Foods are from ARS single nutrient reports, sorted in descending order by nutrient content in terms of common household measures. F ood items and weights in the single nutrient repor ts are adapted from those in 2002 re vision of USDA Home and Garden Bulletin No. 72, Nutritive Value of Foods. Mixed dishes and multiple preparations of the s ame food item have been omitted from this table.

Appendix B2. Food Sources of Vitamin E

Food Sources of Vitamin E ranked by milligrams of vitamin E per standard amount; also calories in the standard amount. (All provide > 10% of RDA for vitamin E for adults, which is 1 5 mg ⟨–tocopherol [AT]/T]/day.)

Food, Standard Amount	AT (mg)	Calories
Fortified ready-to-eat cereals, ~ 1 oz	1.6–12.8	90–107
Sunflower seeds, dry roasted, 1 oz	7.4	165
Almonds, 1 oz	7.3	164
Sunflower oil, high linoleic, 1 Tbsp	5.6	120
Cottonseed oil, 1 Tbsp	4.8	120
Safflower oil, high oleic, 1 Tbsp	4.6	120
Hazelnuts (filberts), 1 oz	4.3	178
Mixed nuts, dry roasted, 1 oz	3.1	168
Turnip greens, frozen, cooked, ½ cup	2.9	24
Tomato paste, ¼ cup	2.8	54
Pine nuts, 1 oz	2.6	191
Peanut butter, 2 Tbsp	2.5	192
Tomato puree, ½ cup	2.5	48
Tomato sauce, ½ cup	2.5	39
Canola oil, 1 Tbsp	2.4	124
Wheat germ, toasted, plain, 2 Tbsp	2.3	54
Peanuts, 1 oz	2.2	166
Avocado, raw, ½ avocado	2.1	161
Carrot juice, canned, ¾ cup	2.1	71
Peanut oil, 1 Tbsp	2.1	119
Corn oil, 1 Tbsp	1.9	120
Olive oil, 1 Tbsp	1.9	119
Spinach, cooked, ½ cup	1.9	21
Dandelion greens, cooked, ½ cup	1.8	18
Sardine, Atlantic, in oil, drained, 3 oz	1.7	177
Blue crab, cooked/canned, 3 oz	1.6	84
Brazil nuts, 1 oz	1.6	186
Herring, Atlantic, pickled, 3 oz	1.5	222

Source: Nutrient values from Agricultural Research Ser vice (ARS) Nutrient Database for Standard Reference, Release 17. Foods are from ARS single nutrient reports, sorted in descending order by nutrient content in terms of common household measures. F ood items and weights in the single nutrient repor ts are adapted from those in 2002 re vision of USDA Home and Garden Bulletin No. 72, Nutritive Value of Foods. Mixed dishes and multiple preparations of the s ame food item have been omitted from this table.

Appendix B3. Food Sources of Iron

Food Sources of Iron ranked by milligrams of iron per standard amount; also calories in the standard amount. (All are > 10% of RDA for teen and adult females, which is 18 8 mg/day.)

Food, Standard Amount	Iron (mg)	Calories
Clams, canned, drained, 3 oz	23.8	126
Fortified ready-to-eat cereals (various), ~ 1 oz	1.8 –21.1	54–127
Oysters, eastern, wild, cooked, moist heat, 3 oz	10.2	116
Organ meats (liver, giblets), various, cooked, 3 oz [a]	5.2–9.9	134–235
Fortified instant cooked cereals (various), 1 packet	4.9–8.1	Varies
Soybeans, mature, cooked, ½ cup	4.4	149
Pumpkin and squash seed kernels, roasted, 1 oz	4.2	148
White beans, canned, ½ cup	3.9	153
Blackstrap molasses, 1 Tbsp	3.5	47
Lentils, cooked, ½ cup	3.3	115
Spinach, cooked from fresh, ½ cup	3.2	21
Beef, chuck, blade roast, lean, cooked, 3 oz	3.1	215
Beef, bottom round, lean, 0″ fat, all grades, cooked, 3 oz	2.8	182
Kidney beans, cooked, ½ cup	2.6	112
Sardines, canned in oil, drained, 3 oz	2.5	177
Beef, rib, lean, ¼″ fat, all grades, cooked, 3 oz	2.4	195
Chickpeas, cooked, ½ cup	2.4	134
Duck, meat only, roasted, 3 oz	2.3	171
Lamb, shoulder, arm, lean, ¼″ fat, choice, cooked, 3 oz	2.3	237
Prune juice, ¾ cup	2.3	136
Shrimp, canned, 3 oz	2.3	102
Cowpeas, cooked, ½ cup	2.2	100
Ground beef, 15% fat, cooked, 3 oz	2.2	212
Tomato puree, ½ cup	2.2	48
Lima beans, cooked, ½ cup	2.2	108
Soybeans, green, cooked, ½ cup	2.2	127
Navy beans, cooked, ½ cup	2.1	127
Refried beans, ½ cup	2.1	118
Beef, top sirloin, lean, 0″ fat, all grades, cooked, 3 oz	2.0	156
Tomato paste, ¼ cup	2.0	54

a High in cholesterol.

Source: Nutrient values from Agricultural Research Ser vice (ARS) Nutrient Database for Standard Reference, Release 17. Foods are from ARS single nutrient reports, sorted in descending order by nutrient content in terms of common household measures. F ood items and weights in the single nutrient repor ts are adapted from those in 2002 re vision of USDA Home and Garden Bulletin No. 72, Nutritive Value of Foods. Mixed dishes and multiple preparations of the s ame food item have been omitted from this table.

Appendix B4. NonDairy Food Sources of Calcium

NonDairy Food Sources of Calcium ranked by milligrams of calcium per standard amount; also calories in the standard amount. The bioavailability may vary. (The AI for adults is 1,000 mg/day.)[a]

Food, Standard Amount	Calcium (mg)	Calories
Fortified ready-to-eat cereals (various), 1 oz	236–1043	88–106
Soy beverage, calcium fortified, 1 cup	368	98
Sardines, Atlantic, in oil, drained, 3 oz	325	177
Tofu, firm, prepared with nigari[b], ½ cup	253	88
Pink salmon, canned, with bone, 3 oz	181	118
Collards, cooked from frozen, ½ cup	178	31
Molasses, blackstrap, 1 Tbsp	172	47
Spinach, cooked from frozen, ½ cup	146	30
Soybeans, green, cooked, ½ cup	130	127
Turnip greens, cooked from frozen, ½ cup	124	24
Ocean perch, Atlantic, cooked, 3 oz	116	103
Oatmeal, plain and flavored, instant, fortified, 1 packet prepared	99–110	97–157
Cowpeas, cooked, ½ cup	106	80
White beans, canned, ½ cup	96	153
Kale, cooked from frozen, ½ cup	90	20
Okra, cooked from frozen, ½ cup	88	26
Soybeans, mature, cooked, ½ cup	88	149
Blue crab, canned, 3 oz	86	84
Beet greens, cooked from fresh, ½ cup	82	19
Pak-choi, Chinese cabbage, cooked from fresh, ½ cup	79	10
Clams, canned, 3 oz	78	126
Dandelion greens, cooked from fresh, ½ cup	74	17
Rainbow trout, farmed, cooked, 3 oz	73	144

[a] Both calcium content and bioavailability should be considered when selecting dietar y sources of calcium. Some plant foods have calcium that is well absorbed, but the large quantity of plant foods that would be needed to provide as much calcium as in a glass of milk may be unachie vable for many. Many other calciumfortified foods are available, but the percentage of calcium that can be absorbed is unavailable for many of them.

[b] Calcium sulfate and magnesium chloride.

Source: Nutrient values from Agricultural Research Ser vice (ARS) Nutrient Database for Standard Reference, Release 17. Foods are from ARS single nutrient reports, sorted in descending order by nutrient content in terms of common household measures. F ood items and weights in the single nutrient repor ts are adapted from those in 2002 re vision of USDA Home and Garden Bulletin No. 72, Nutritive Value of Foods. Mixed dishes and multiple preparations of the s ame food item have been omitted from this table.

Appendix B5. Food Sources of Calcium

Food Sources of Calcium ranked by milligrams of calcium per standard amount; also calories in the standard amount. (All are > 20% of AI for adults 1950, which is 1,000 ,000 mg/day.)

Food, Standard Amount	Calcium (mg)	Calories
Plain yogurt, non-fat (13 g protein/8 oz), 8-oz container	452	127
Romano cheese, 1.5 oz	452	165
Pasteurized process Swiss cheese, 2 oz	438	190
Plain yogurt, low-fat (12 g protein/8 oz), 8-oz container	415	143
Fruit yogurt, low-fat (10 g protein/8 oz), 8-oz container	345	232
Swiss cheese, 1.5 oz	336	162
Ricotta cheese, part skim, ½ cup	335	170
Pasteurized process American cheese food, 2 oz	323	188
Provolone cheese, 1.5 oz	321	150
Mozzarella cheese, part-skim, 1.5 oz	311	129
Cheddar cheese, 1.5 oz	307	171
Fat-free (skim) milk, 1 cup	306	83
Muenster cheese, 1.5 oz	305	156
1% low-fat milk, 1 cup	290	102
Low-fat chocolate milk (1%), 1 cup	288	158
2% reduced fat milk, 1 cup	285	122
Reduced fat chocolate milk (2%), 1 cup	285	180
Buttermilk, low-fat, 1 cup	284	98
Chocolate milk, 1 cup	280	208
Whole milk, 1 cup	276	146
Yogurt, plain, whole milk (8 g protein/8 oz), 8-oz container	275	138
Ricotta cheese, whole milk, ½ cup	255	214
Blue cheese, 1.5 oz	225	150
Mozzarella cheese, whole milk, 1.5 oz	215	128
Feta cheese, 1.5 oz	210	113

Source: Nutrient values from Agricultural Research Ser vice (ARS) Nutrient Database for Standard Reference, Release 17. Foods are from ARS single nutrient reports, sorted in descending order by nutrient content in terms of common household measures. F ood items and weights in the single nutrient repor ts are adapted from those in 2002 re vision of USDA Home and Garden Bulletin No. 72, Nutritive Value of Foods. Mixed dishes and multiple preparations of the s ame food item have been omitted from this table.

Appendix B6. Food Sources of Vitamin A

Food Sources of Vitamin A ranked by micrograms Retinol Activity Equivalents (R AE) of vitamin A per standard amount; also calories in the standard amount. (All are > 20% of RDA for adult men, which is 9 00 mg/day RAE.)

Food, Standard Amount	Vitamin A (μg RAE)	Calories
Organ meats (liver, giblets), various, cooked, 3 oz[a]	1490–9126	134–235
Carrot juice, ¾ cup	1692	71
Sweetpotato with peel, baked, 1 medium	1096	103
Pumpkin, canned, ½ cup	953	42
Carrots, cooked from fresh, ½ cup	671	27
Spinach, cooked from frozen, ½ cup	573	30
Collards, cooked from frozen, ½ cup	489	31
Kale, cooked from frozen, ½ cup	478	20
Mixed vegetables, canned, ½ cup	474	40
Turnip greens, cooked from frozen, ½ cup	441	24
Instant cooked cereals, fortified, prepared, 1 packet	285–376	75–97
Various ready-to-eat cereals, with added vit. A, ~ 1 oz	180–376	100–117
Carrot, raw, 1 small	301	20
Beet greens, cooked, ½ cup	276	19
Winter squash, cooked, ½ cup	268	38
Dandelion greens, cooked, ½ cup	260	18
Cantaloupe, raw, ¼ medium melon	233	46
Mustard greens, cooked, ½ cup	221	11
Pickled herring, 3 oz	219	222
Red sweet pepper, cooked, ½ cup	186	19
Chinese cabbage, cooked, ½ cup	180	10

a High in cholesterol.

Source: Nutrient values from Agricultural Research Ser vice (ARS) Nutrient Database for Standard Reference, Release 17. Foods are from ARS single nutrient reports, sorted in descending order by nutrient content in terms of common household measures. F ood items and weights in the single nutrient repor ts are adapted from those in 2002 re vision of USDA Home and Garden Bulletin No. 72, Nutritive Value of Foods. Mixed dishes and multiple preparations of the s ame food item have been omitted from this table.

Appendix B7. Food Sources of Magnesium

Food Sources of Magnesium ranked by milligrams of magnesium per standard amount; also calories in the standard amount.(All are > 10% of RDA DA for adult men, which is 420 mg/day .)

Food, Standard Amount	Magnesium (mg)	Calories
Pumpkin and squash seed kernels, roasted, 1 oz	151	148
Brazil nuts, 1 oz	107	186
Bran ready-to-eat cereal (100%), ~1 oz	103	74
Halibut, cooked, 3 oz	91	119
Quinoa, dry, ¼ cup	89	159
Spinach, canned, ½ cup	81	25
Almonds, 1 oz	78	164
Spinach, cooked from fresh, ½ cup	78	20
Buckwheat flour, ¼ cup	75	101
Cashews, dry roasted, 1 oz	74	163
Soybeans, mature, cooked, ½ cup	74	149
Pine nuts, dried, 1 oz	71	191
Mixed nuts, oil roasted, with peanuts, 1 oz	67	175
White beans, canned, ½ cup	67	154
Pollock, walleye, cooked, 3 oz	62	96
Black beans, cooked, ½ cup	60	114
Bulgur, dry, ¼ cup	57	120
Oat bran, raw, ¼ cup	55	58
Soybeans, green, cooked, ½ cup	54	127
Tuna, yellowfin, cooked, 3 oz	54	118
Artichokes (hearts), cooked, ½ cup	50	42
Peanuts, dry roasted, 1 oz	50	166
Lima beans, baby, cooked from frozen, ½ cup	50	95
Beet greens, cooked, ½ cup	49	19
Navy beans, cooked, ½ cup	48	127
Tofu, firm, prepared with nigari[a], ½ cup	47	88
Okra, cooked from frozen, ½ cup	47	26
Soy beverage, 1 cup	47	127
Cowpeas, cooked, ½ cup	46	100
Hazelnuts, 1 oz	46	178
Oat bran muffin, 1 oz	45	77
Great northern beans, cooked, ½ cup	44	104
Oat bran, cooked, ½ cup	44	44
Buckwheat groats, roasted, cooked, ½ cup	43	78
Brown rice, cooked, ½ cup	42	108
Haddock, cooked, 3 oz	42	95

a Calcium sulfate and magnesium chloride.

Source: Nutrient values from Agricultural Research Ser vice (ARS) Nutrient Database for Standard Reference, Release 17. Foods are from ARS single nutrient reports, sorted in descending order by nutrient content in terms of common household measures. F ood items and weights in the single nutrient repor ts are adapted from those in 2002 re vision of USDA Home and Garden Bulletin No. 72, Nutritive Value of Foods. Mixed dishes and multiple preparations of the s ame food item have been omitted from this table.

Appendix B8. Food Sources of Dietary Fiber

Food Sources of Dietary Fiber ranked by grams of dietary fiber per standard amount; also calories in the standard amount. (All are >10% of AI for adult women, which is 25 grams/day .)

Food, Standard Amount	Dietary Fiber (g)	Calories
Navy beans, cooked, ½ cup	9.5	128
Bran ready-to-eat cereal (100%), ½ cup	8.8	78
Kidney beans, canned, ½ cup	8.2	109
Split peas, cooked, ½ cup	8.1	116
Lentils, cooked, ½ cup	7.8	115
Black beans, cooked, ½ cup	7.5	114
Pinto beans, cooked, ½ cup	7.7	122
Lima beans, cooked, ½ cup	6.6	108
Artichoke, globe, cooked, 1 each	6.5	60
White beans, canned, ½ cup	6.3	154
Chickpeas, cooked, ½ cup	6.2	135
Great northern beans, cooked, ½ cup	6.2	105
Cowpeas, cooked, ½ cup	5.6	100
Soybeans, mature, cooked, ½ cup	5.2	149
Bran ready-to-eat cereals, various, ~1 oz	2.6–5.0	90–108
Crackers, rye wafers, plain, 2 wafers	5.0	74
Sweetpotato, baked, with peel, 1 medium (146 g)	4.8	131
Asian pear, raw, 1 small	4.4	51
Green peas, cooked, ½ cup	4.4	67
Whole-wheat English muffin, 1 each	4.4	134
Pear, raw, 1 small	4.3	81
Bulgur, cooked, ½ cup	4.1	76
Mixed vegetables, cooked, ½ cup	4.0	59
Raspberries, raw, ½ cup	4.0	32
Sweetpotato, boiled, no peel, 1 medium (156 g)	3.9	119
Blackberries, raw, ½ cup	3.8	31
Potato, baked, with skin, 1 medium	3.8	161
Soybeans, green, cooked, ½ cup	3.8	127
Stewed prunes, ½ cup	3.8	133
Figs, dried, ¼ cup	3.7	93
Dates, ¼ cup	3.6	126
Oat bran, raw, ¼ cup	3.6	58
Pumpkin, canned, ½ cup	3.6	42
Spinach, frozen, cooked, ½ cup	3.5	30
Shredded wheat ready-to-eat cereals, various, ~1 oz	2.8–3.4	96
Almonds, 1 oz	3.3	164
Apple with skin, raw, 1 medium	3.3	72
Brussels sprouts, frozen, cooked, ½ cup	3.2	33
Whole-wheat spaghetti, cooked, ½ cup	3.1	87

Appendix B8: Continued

Food, Standard Amount	Dietary Fiber (g)	Calories
Banana, 1 medium	3.1	105
Orange, raw, 1 medium	3.1	62
Oat bran muffin, 1 small	3.0	178
Guava, 1 medium	3.0	37
Pearled barley, cooked, ½ cup	3.0	97
Sauerkraut, canned, solids, and liquids, ½ cup	3.0	23
Tomato paste, ¼ cup	2.9	54
Winter squash, cooked, ½ cup	2.9	38
Broccoli, cooked, ½ cup	2.8	26
Parsnips, cooked, chopped, ½ cup	2.8	55
Turnip greens, cooked, ½ cup	2.5	15
Collards, cooked, ½ cup	2.7	25
Okra, frozen, cooked, ½ cup	2.6	26
Peas, edible-podded, cooked, ½ cup	2.5	42

Source: ARS Nutrient Database for Standard Reference, Release 17. Foods are from single nutrient repor ts, which are sorted either by food description or in descending order by nutrient content in terms of common household measures. The food items and weights in these repor ts are adapted from those in 2002 re vision of USDA Home and Garden Bulletin No. 72, Nutritive Value of Foods. Mixed dishes and multiple preparations of the s ame food item have been omitted.

Appendix B9. Food Sources of Vitamin C

Food Sources of Vitamin C ranked by milligrams of vitamin C per standard amount; also calories in the standard amount. (All provide > 20% of RDA for adult men, which is 9 0 mg/day.)

Food, Standard Amount	Vitamin C (mg)	Calories
Guava, raw, ½ cup	188	56
Red sweet pepper, raw, ½ cup	142	20
Red sweet pepper, cooked, ½ cup	116	19
Kiwi fruit, 1 medium	70	46
Orange, raw, 1 medium	70	62
Orange juice, ¾ cup	61–93	79–84
Green pepper, sweet, raw, ½ cup	60	15
Green pepper, sweet, cooked, ½ cup	51	19
Grapefruit juice, ¾ cup	50–70	71–86
Vegetable juice cocktail, ¾ cup	50	34
Strawberries, raw, ½ cup	49	27
Brussels sprouts, cooked, ½ cup	48	28
Cantaloupe, ¼ medium	47	51
Papaya, raw, ¼ medium	47	30
Kohlrabi, cooked, ½ cup	45	24
Broccoli, raw, ½ cup	39	15
Edible pod peas, cooked, ½ cup	38	34
Broccoli, cooked, ½ cup	37	26
Sweetpotato, canned, ½ cup	34	116
Tomato juice, ¾ cup	33	31
Cauliflower, cooked, ½ cup	28	17
Pineapple, raw, ½ cup	28	37
Kale, cooked, ½ cup	27	18
Mango, ½ cup	23	54

Source: Nutrient values from Agricultural Research Ser vice (ARS) Nutrient Database for Standard Reference, Release 17. Foods are from ARS single nutrient reports, sorted in descending order by nutrient content in terms of common household measures. F ood items and weights in the single nutrient repor ts are adapted from those in 2002 re vision of USDA Home and Garden Bulletin No. 72, Nutritive Value of Foods. Mixed dishes and multiple preparations of the s ame food item have been omitted from this table.

APPENDIX C. GLOSSARY OF TERMS

Acceptable Macronutrient Distribution Ranges (AMDR) – Range of intake for a particular energy source that is associated with reduced risk of chronic disease while providing intakes of essential nutrients. If an individual consumes in excess of the AMDR, there is a potential of increasing the risk of chronic diseases and/or insufficient intakes of essential nutrients.

Added Sugars – processing or preparation. Added sugars do not include naturally occurring sugars such as those that occur in milk and fruits.

Adequate Intakes (AI) – A recommended average daily nutrient intake level based on observed or experimentally determined approximations or esti- mates of mean nutrient intake by a group (or groups) of apparently healthy people. The AI is used when the Estimated Average Requirement cannot be determined.

Basic Food Groups – groups are grains; fruits; vegetables; milk, yogurt, and cheese; and meat, poultry, fish, dried peas and beans, eggs, and nuts. In the DAS H Eating Plan, nuts, seeds, and dry beans are a separate food group from meat, poultry, fish, and eggs.

Body Mass Index (BMI) – BMI is a practical measure for approximating total body fat and is a measure of weight in relation to height. It is calculated as weight in kilograms divided by the square of the height in meters.

Cardiovascular Disease – Refers to diseases of the heart and diseases of the blood vessel system (arteries, capillaries, veins) within a person's entire body, such as the brain, legs, and lungs.

Cholesterol – sterol present in all animal tissues. Free cholesterol is a component of cell membranes and serves as a precursor for steroid hormones, including estrogen, testosterone, aldosterone, and bile acids. Humans are able to synthesize sufficient cholesterol to meet biologic require - ments, and there is no evidence for a dietary requirement for cholesterol.

- **Dietary cholesterol** – Consumed from foods of animal origin, including meat, fish, poultry, eggs, and dairy products. Plant foods, such as grains, fruits and vegetables, and oils from these sources contain no dietary cholesterol.
- **Serum cholesterol** – both lipids and proteins. Three major classes of lipoproteins are found in the serum of a fasting individual: low-density lipoprotein (LDL), high-density lipoprotein (HDL), and very-low-density

lipoprotein (VLDL). Another lipoprotein class, intermediate-density lipoprotein (IDL), resides between VLDL and LDL; in clinical practice, IDL is included in the LDL measurement.

Chronic Diseases – Range of intake leading causes of death and disability in the United States. These diseases account for 7 of every 10 deaths and affect the quality of life of 90 million Americans. Although chronic diseases are among the most common and costly health problems, they are also among the most preventable. Adopting healthy behaviors such as eating nutritious foods, being physically Sugars and syrups that are added to foods during active, and avoiding tobacco use can prevent or control the devastating effects of these diseases.

Coronary Heart Disease – A narrowing of the small blood vessels that A recommended average daily nutrient intake level supply blood and oxygen to the heart (coronary arteries).

Daily Food Intake Pattern – Identifies the types and amounts of foods that are recommended to be eaten each day and that meet specific nutritional goals. (*Federal Register Notice* , vol. 68, no. 176, p. 53536, Thursday, September 11, 2003)

Danger Zone – The temperature that allows bacteria to multiply rapidly and produce toxins, between 40°F and 140 F. To keep food out of this danger zone, keep cold food cold and hot food hot. Keep food cold in the refriger- ator, in coolers, or on ice in the service line. Keep hot food in the oven, in heated chafing dishes, or in preheated steam tables, warming trays, and/or slow cookers. Never leave perishable foods, such as meat, poultry, eggs, and casseroles, in the danger zone longer than 2 hours or longer than 1 hour in temperatures above 90°F

Dietary Fiber – Nonstarch polysaccharides and lignin that are not digested by enzymes in the small intestine. Dietary fiber typically refers to nondi- gestable carbohydrates from plant foods.

Dietary Reference Intakes (DRIs) – A set of nutrient-based reference values that expand upon and replace the former Recommended Dietary Allowances (RDAs) in the United States and the Recommended Nutrient Intakes (RNIs) in Canada. They are actually a set of four reference values: Estimated Average Requirements (EARs), RDAs, AIs, and Tolerable Upper Intake Levels (ULs).

Discretionary Calorie Allowance – The balance of calories remaining in a person's energy allowance after accounting for the number of calories needed to meet recommended nutrient intakes through consumption of foods in low-fat or no added sugar forms. The discretionary calorie allowance may be used in selecting forms of foods that are not the most nutrient-dense (e.g., whole milk rather than fat-free milk) or may be addi- tions to foods (e.g., salad dressing, sugar, butter).

Energy Allowance – A person's energy allowance is the calorie intake at which weight maintenance occurs.

Estimated Average Requirements – EAR is the average daily nutrient intake level estimated to meet the requirement of half the healthy individuals in a particular life stage and gender group.

Estimated Energy Requirement – The EER represents the average dietary energy intake that will maintain energy balance in a healthy person of a given gender, age, weight, height, and physical activity level.

FDAMA – The Food and Drug Administration Modernization Act, enacted Nov. 21, 1997, amended the Federal Food, Drug, and Cosmetic Act relating to the regulation of food, drugs, devices, and biological products. With the passage of FDAMA, Congress enhanced FDA's mission in ways that recog- nized the Agency would be operating in a 21st century characterized by increasing technological, trade, and public health complexities.

FightBAC! – A national public education campaign to promote food safety to consumers and educate them on how to handle and prepare food safely. In this campaign, pathogens are represented by a cartoon-like bacteria char- acter named "BAC".

Foodborne Disease – Caused by consuming contaminated foods or bever- ages. Many different disease-causing microbes, or pathogens, can contaminate foods, so there are many different foodborne infections. In addition, poisonous chemicals, or other harmful substances, can cause foodborne diseases if they are present in food. The most commonly recog- nized foodborne infections are those caused by the bacteria *Campylobacter, Salmonella,* and *E. coli* O157:H7, and by a group of viruses called calicivirus, also known as the Norwalk and Norwalk-like viruses.

Heme Iron – One of two forms of iron occurring in foods. Heme Iron is bound within the iron-carrying proteins (hemoglobin and myoglobin) found in meat, poultry, and fish. While it contributes a smaller portion of iron to typical American diets than non-heme iron, a larger proportion of heme iron is absorbed.

High Fructose Corn Syrup (HFCS) – A corn sweetener derived from the wet milling of corn. Cornstarch is converted to a syrup that is nearly all dex trose. HFCS is found in numerous foods and beverages on the grocery store shelves.

Hydrogenation – A chemical reaction that adds hydrogen atoms in an unsaturated fat, thus saturating it and making it solid at room temperature.

Leisure-Time Physical Activity – Physical activity that is performed during exercise, recreation, or any additional time other than that associated with one's regular job duties, occupation, or transportation.

Listeriosis – A serious infection caused by eating food contaiminated with the bacterium *Listeria monocytogenes*, which has recently been recognized as an important public health problem in the United States. The disease affects primarily pregnant women, their fetuses, newborns, and adults with weakened immune systems. Listeria is killed by pasteurization and cooking; however, in certain ready-to-eat foods, such as hot dogs and deli meats, contamination may occur after cooking/manufacture but before packaging. *Listeria monocytogenes* can survive at refrigerated temperatures.

Macronutrient – The dietary macronutrient groups are carbohydrates, proteins, and fats.

Micronutrient – Vitamins and minerals that are required in the human diet in very small amounts.

Moderate Physical Activity – Any activity that burns 3.5 to 7 kcal/min or the equivalent of 3 to 6 metabolic equivalents (M ETs) and results in achieving 60 to 73 percent of peak heart rate. An estimate of a person's age from 220. Examples of moderate physical activity include walking briskly, mowing the lawn, dancing, swimming, or bicycling on level terrain. A person should feel some exertion but should be able to carry on a conversation comfort- ably during the activity.

Monounsaturated Fatty Acids – Monounsaturated fatty acids (MUFAs) have one double bond. Plant sources that are rich in MUFAs include vegetable oils (e.g., canola oil, olive oil, high oleic s afflower and sunflower oils) that are liquid at room temperature and nuts.

Nutrient – Dense Foods – substantial amounts of vitamins and minerals and relatively fewer calories.

Ounce – Equivalent One of two forms — of iron occurring in foods. Heme iron is as equal to a one-ounce slice of bread; in the meat, poultry, fish, dry beans, eggs, and nuts food group, the amount of food counted as equal to one ounce of cooked meat, poultry, or fish. Examples are listed in table 1 and appendix A-1.

n-6 PUFAs – A corn sweetener derived from the wet be synthesized by humans and, therefore, is considered essential in the diet. Primary sources are liquid vegetable oils, including soybean oil, corn oil, and safflower oil.

n-3 PUFAs – α-linolenic acid is an n-3 fatty acid that is required because it is not synthesized by humans and, therefore, is considered essential in the diet. Physical activity that is performed during It is obtained from plant sources, including soybean oil, canola oil, walnuts, and flaxseed. Eicosapentaenoic acid (EPA) and docosahexaenoic acid (DHA) regular job duties, occupation, or transportation. are long chain n-3 fatty acids that are contained in fish and shellfish.

Pathogen – Any microorganism that can cause or is capable of causing disease.

Polyunsaturated Fatty Acids Polyunsaturated fatty acids (PUFAs) have two or more double bonds and may be of two types, based on the position of the first double bond.

Portion Size – The amount of a food consumed in one eating occasion.

Recommended Dietary Allowance (RDA) – The dietary intake level that is sufficient to meet the nutrient requirement of nearly all (97 to 98 percent) healthy individuals in a particular life stage and gender group.

Resistance Exercise – Anaerobic training, including weight training, weight machine use, and resistance band workouts. Resistance training will increase strength, muscular endurance, and muscle size, while running and jogging will not.
Saturated Fatty Acids—Saturated fatty acids have no double bonds. They primarily come from animal products such as meat and dairy products. In general, animal fats are solid at room temperature.

Sedentary Behaviors – In scientific literature, sedentary is often defined in terms of little or no physical activity during leisure time. A sedentar y lifestyle is a lifestyle characterized by little or no physical activity.

Serving Size – A standardized amount of a food, such as a cup or an ounce, used in providing dietar y guidance or in making comparisons among similar foods.
Tolerable Upper Intake Level (UL) – The highest average daily nutrient intake level likely to pose no risk of adverse health affects for nearly all indi- viduals in a particular life stage and gender group. As intake increases above the UL, the potential risk of adverse health affects increases.

Trans **fatty acids** – *Trans* fatty acids, or *trans* fats, are unsaturated fatty acids that contain at least one non-conjugated double bond in the *trans* configu- ration. Sources of *trans* fatty acids include hydrogenated/partially hydrogenated vegetable oils that are used to make shortening and commer- cially prepared baked goods, snack foods, fried foods, and margarine. *Trans* fatty acids also are present in foods that come from ruminant animals (e.g., cattle and sheep). Such foods include dairy products, beef, and lamb.

Vegetarian – There are several categories of vegetarians, all of whom avoid meat and/or animal products. The vegan or total vegetarian diet includes only foods from plants: fruits, vegetables, legumes (dried beans and peas), grains, seeds, and nuts. The lactovegetarian diet includes plant foods plus cheese and other dairy products. The ovo-lactovegetarian (or lacto-ovovege- tarian) diet also includes eggs. Semi-vegetarians do not eat red meat but include chicken and fish with plant foods, dairy products, and eggs.

Vigorous Physical Activity – Any activity that burns more that 7 kcal/min or the equivalent of 6 or more metabolic equivalents (METs) and results in achieving 74 to 88 percent of peak heart rate. An estimate of a person's peak heart rate can be obtained by subtracting the person's age from 220. Examples of vigorous physical activity include jogging, mowing the lawn with a nonmotorized push mower, chopping wood, participating in high- impact aerobic dancing, swimming continuous laps, or bicycling uphill. Vigorous-intensity physical activity may be intense enough to represent a substantial challenge to an individual and results in a significant increase in heart and breathing rate.

Weight-Bearing Exercise – Any activity one performs that works bones and muscles against gravity, including walking, running, hiking, dancing, g ymnas- tics, and soccer.

Whole Grains – Foods made from the entire grain seed, usually called the kernel, which consists of the bran, germ, and endosperm. If the kernel has been cracked, crushed, or flaked, it must retain nearly the same relative proportions of bran, germ, and endosperm as the original grain in order to be called whole grain.[1]

REFERENCES

[1]   AACC Press Release, AACC To Create Consumer-Friendly Whole Grain Definition, March 5, 2004. http://www.aaccnet.org/news/CFWholeGrain.asp.

Appendix D. Acronyms

AI— Adequate Intakes

AMDR— Acceptable Macronutrient Distribution Range

ARS— Agricultural Research Service

BMI— Body Mass Index

CSFII— Continuing Survey of Food Intakes by Individuals

DASH— Dietary Approaches to Stop Hypertension

DFE— Dietary Folate Equivalent

DHA— Docosahexaenoic acid

DRI— Dietary Reference Intake

DV— Daily Value

EAR— Estimated Average Requirement

EER— Estimated Energy Requirement

EPA— Eicosapentaenoic acid

FDA— Food and Drug Administration

FDAMA— Food and Drug Administration Modernization Act

HDL— High-density lipoprotein

HHS— U.S. Department of Health and Human Services

IU— International unit

LDL— Low-density lipoprotein

RAE— Retinol Activity Equivalent

RDA— Recommended Dietar y Allowance

USDA— U.S. Department of Agriculture

INDEX

Index